© 2015 Asa Ka....

The information in this book is for educational purposes only, it is not intended to be a substitute for professional medical advice.

This book is for you Freja, my daughter, my love, my everything.

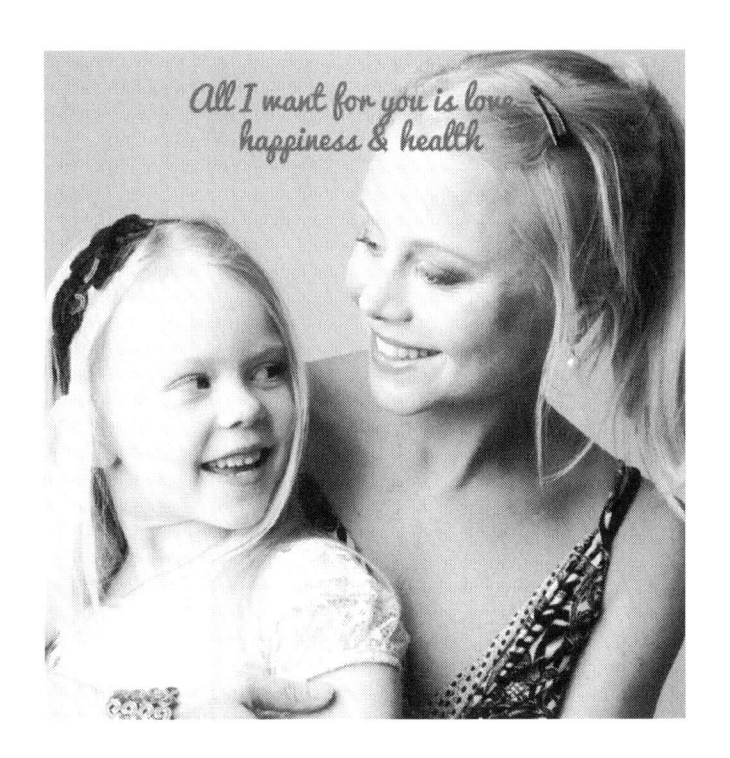

Chapters

Part One

1. PREFACE
2. WHO AM I? AND WHAT'S PPP GOT TO DO WITH IT?
3. WHAT IS PPP?
4. PPP – WHAT CAN A CASE STUDY TELL US?
5. TODAY'S MEDICAL TREATMENT OF PPP – POTIONS AND LOTIONS
6. PPP AND ME
7. UNDERSTANDING THE IMMUNE SYSTEM
8. THE GUT AND ITS INHABITANTS
9. ANTIBIOTICS
10. BACTERIAL BIOFILMS
11. YEAST INFECTIONS
12. GLUTEN
13. LEAKY GUT SYNDROME
14. CROSS REACTIVITY
15. STRESS / How stress affects our digestion and general health

Part Two

16. WHAT TRIGGERS PPP? / Getting to the Root of the Situation
17. SIX STEPS TO TREAT PPP
18. HOW TO IMPROVE YOUR IMMUNE SYSTEM THROUGH DIET
19. ALPHABET SOUP: AN OVERVIEW OF SPECIFIC DIETS – GAPS, PALEO, HCFC, FODMAP AND MORE
20. SUPPLEMENTS – THE HOWS AND WHYS
21. FINAL THOUGHTS…
22. RESOURCES

"The natural healing force within each of us is the greatest force in getting well."
— Hippocrates

Part 1

PREFACE

Congratulations on picking this book and giving me a chance to help you treat your **Palmoplantar Pustular Psoriasis (PPP)** naturally.

I have been through the same painful and lonely journey as you, but have now thankfully been symptom-free for the last three years. Before that I was ill and in daily pain, my skin oozing, my body was ravaged by a life-destroying disease. My family felt it the most – for them, watching a loved one constantly hurting was heartbreaking.

There are no words to describe how absolutely amazing life can feel after coming out the end of a very dark tunnel, not only for me but also for my family. This illness affects every aspect of your life – the ability to use your hands and walk properly, your mental health, even your sex life. I'm glad my daughter was only a toddler at the time of my illness and has no clear memories of that period.

I wrote this book as I was frustrated with the absence of information about PPP and the lack of understanding by the many doctors I encountered while I was sick. I'm compelled to help other sufferers who may be in the same situation as I've been. I understand how hopeless and depressed you feel during the repeated outbreaks of this disease, as your hands and feet are racked by itchiness and pain; and how self-conscious you feel as skin erupts in pustules and fissures. I understand, and I can help.

I have spent thousands of hours gathering information on PPP, trying to find ways and solutions to heal. I have since completed a course and received a diploma in nutrition, and from my research and studies I know nutrition is the key to heal from any autoimmune disease.

This book is written as a framework to help you understand how the immune system works and what type of disease PPP is, and what you need to do to get your life back. I want to show you how, with just a few lifestyle changes, you are able to recover.

It doesn't matter if you have recently been diagnosed or if you had the disease for years, the most important thing is to understand the healing process takes time. The body is complex and we are all different, what might work for some might not work for others. Personally, it took me over two months to heal completely, so you need to give yourself and your body time to heal.

There are several conventional treatments to control PPP; I will mention them in this book as well, but my aim is to show you how to treat this condition naturally without autoimmune suppressants such as biologics and other drugs.

PPP is a complex illness. I'll provide an overview about what's happening inside your body and why you got sick in the first place, then discuss what you need to do to recover and how to build a functional immune system again. You can do this through optimal nutrition and addressing the root causes of the disease.

I have divided the book in two parts. In the first part I discuss how the immune system works and what causes it to stop functioning, and how this change in function eventually leads to an autoimmune disease. In the second part the focus is on how to repair your immune system.

I am so happy you have chosen to take your health into your own hands and you have given me a chance to help you along your journey to recovery.

You are welcome to visit my blog and connect with me at www.well-healed.com

All the best,

Åsa x

WHO AM I? AND WHAT'S PPP GOT TO DO WITH IT?

As I type this I will soon turn 38 years old; I'm a woman in my prime who is trying to live life to the fullest. I have a daughter who is nearly seven and I'm married to an Irish man who just happens to be the best husband and father in the world.

We're currently located in my hometown of Gothenburg, Sweden, we moved here shortly after my daughter was born in Ireland. I work full-time for a Swedish international company and I'm probably working too much, but life is generally good. We try to travel as whenever possible to see other cultures and to experience the world.

I spend a lot of my time researching health and lifestyle changes, now one of my main interests. This was not always the case, but it became my calling after being very ill for a number of years.

My life was side-tracked by a strange assortment of symptoms, and eventually after going from doctor-to-doctor, I was told I had an autoimmune disease – **palmoplantar pustular psoriasis (PPP)**.

Before developing PPP my immune system had gradually declined over the last couple of years. About six months after my daughter was born, I always seemed to have a cold, and developed strange skin symptoms. I continually suffered from thrush – a painful infection that understandably affected my love life. My skin got really bad and I developed rosacea, a facial condition where your skin goes red and little spots appeared everywhere. I had a recurring sty on my eye lid and the eyelashes kept falling off.

All of these were warning signs, which I chose to ignore at the time.

Today I know better. My body was trying to tell me something wasn't right and to slow down. I pushed myself too hard in every direction – I wanted to have a successful career, marriage, and family. I tried to be perfect at everything, and failed.

It's a sign of our times, and a fact of modern life; everyone is busy. Convenience – in food, communication, or entertainment – is what's important. Get it now and get it fast. Everything is slickly packaged and ready for consumption. Like food.

Like many of you, I was far too busy. I didn't care about what type of food I put into my body. Food was not on my priority list back then as there was simply no time to prepare nutritious food.

Or, so I thought.

We all set our own priorities. And I soon learned to reprioritize.

After my diagnosis I was shocked to find there was no quick fix. Doctors suggested some lotions and potions, but that was about it. I didn't know much about autoimmune diseases. Neither did the doctors I was seeing.

I had loads of questions but didn't get any answers. The doctors couldn't help me. I already had my five minutes that doctors are scheduled to dedicate to each patient here in Sweden. Off to back home they sent me, ready to deal with the next patient.

I'm an inquisitive person, and some things I just have to know. I need to know the 'hows and whys' before doing something; and I presume you are similar as you're reading this book. When I began doing my research and looking into the causes of this disease, I realized there might be natural ways to combat PPP.

"There is no cure, PPP is for life. You'll never heal, this condition is chronic." I couldn't accept the words of my dermatologist. "You might be lucky and have spells of remission, but you're going to have to learn to live with it." Those words still haunt me.

There might not be a cure, but there is hope.

I agree with doctors that there is no cure. A cure means you can do something that eliminates the problem and the illness will never come back. I don't think that's the case with any disease. Once it's there you will always be receptive to get it again if you do not maintain your body, and remove the root cause. I will use the words remission and heal as synonyms in this book as I know the word 'cure' might be a bit provocative.

Throughout my struggles with PPP, I read, and I learned. I began to understand the science of food and why we eat, as well as the importance of our gut flora. The obvious reason why we eat is to satiate our hunger, but it's also the fuel we need to for our body to function properly. I learned about the foods that do not provide any nourishment to our body, or more specifically, the cells we're composed of. I also learned about the foods that make our bodies thrive.

When I was sick I was so eager to implement various treatments I read about to heal my body. I tried nearly everything through random trial and error. I read about other people's health improving after taking probiotics, so I tried that – with no success. I read that D3 Vitamins are the super vitamin for the immune system, but it had no effect on me, at first. It was after a year of trying different things I eventually learned that healing is not about superficial strategies, like slapping on Band-Aids. You need to understand the whole system to be successful, and make change with the whole system in mind.

Through my studies I sadly came to realize that most doctors have little to no nutritional education. They are taught how to treat a symptom, but not how to change the cause. An autoimmune disease is not one single symptom, but a disease with complex causes and can stem from many factors.

Now, after three years of not having a single outbreak of PPP, I'm confident that my healing system works and I want to help you to heal too. We all have different triggers for the onset of this disease, and you will need to identify your particular triggers to be successful.

I'll walk you through different possible triggers and offer potential solutions. I'm not saying it's going to be easy – you'll need to cut out certain foods you might love and add other ones you may not have considered before. My mission is to help you. This is not a diet plan. Some of you are going to lose weight and for those who are too skinny and would love a couple extra pounds, you'll probably gain some as your body turns toward health. You're not going to starve but will need to break old patterns of bad food choices.

I also want to mention my book is not about curing psoriasis. I don't have any other type of psoriasis issues apart from PPP, which some scientist do not even consider being part of the psoriasis family. I do know if you boost your immune system and remove all the things from your diet that are harming your body, all the other issues you might have will probably go away too. There are a lot of autoimmune diseases, but thankfully one solution that will work on most of them. I will dig deeper in to this later in the chapter on how to repair your immune system.

The good news for most people is that after your body has been restored, you can treat yourself once in a while to foods that are defiantly a no-no during the healing process. And when I write 'once in a while' I mean occasionally at a party or a special occasion. If you indulge in chocolate cake every day, you'll be right back where you started.

We're in this together; let your journey begin to a healthy life without pain and discomfort.

WHAT IS PPP?

When I first was diagnosed with PPP by my dermatologist, I had never heard of it before and had no idea what it was; while at the same time I was happy to finally have a diagnosis and a name for what was wrong with me. After months of not knowing what was going on in my body, and living with the thought I had scabies (I will tell you about this later on in this book), I was thrilled to know that the illness was real and had a name.

The short moment of happiness quickly faded when my doctor informed me the disease is chronic, and would probably be a life-long affliction. The doctor said that if I'm lucky, there will be times of remission. If I'm lucky! And if I was very unlucky there might be times where I'd have to use a wheelchair to get around, as the feet can become very sore after PPP blisters form crusts that crack and bleed. It didn't sound good.

Palmoplantar pustulosis (PPP) goes under a few different names such as **palmoplantar pustular psoriasis**, **pustulosis palmoplantaris**, and **pustulosis**. They all mean the same thing, and in this book I'll use the short form **PPP**.

PPP is a chronic inflammatory illness characterized by accumulation of pustules on the palms and soles that erupt repeatedly over time. It's localized (doesn't spread to other body parts) but is very difficult to treat. It occurs almost mostly in smokers (current or past), and it does not necessarily go away when the patient quits smoking. There is an association with other autoimmune diseases, particularly gluten sensitivity and celiac disease, thyroid disease and type 2 diabetes.

The little blisters or pustules are not contagious but can appear to be to somebody who doesn't know what it is, and esthetically it's not a pretty sight. Red, swollen blisters can turn into yellowish crusts and painful cracks. The condition varies in severity and can persist for many years. It's not known what triggers flare-ups as there are not many studies on the subject, but in a number of studies from different parts of the world, the onset of PPP has been closely linked with cigarette smoking as well as recurrent strep throat infections.

The general medical understanding is that PPP has little effect on the health in general, but can be very uncomfortable. Usually, pressure, rubbing and friction will worsen PPP. I don't agree with the idea that PPP doesn't affect the general health; any autoimmune disease signals there is something very wrong and should be dealt with to avoid any future health issues.

According to some researchers PPP is part of the psoriasis family, and to others it is not. The views differ as the genetic predispositions are not the same for the both psoriasis and PPP.

The crops of pustules may occur with psoriasis, or like in my case without any other skin disease (apart from the rosacea on my face). The disease is very uncommon and there are no available data of how much of the general population is affected. The Swedish dermatology department have an outpatient data register which found an incidence of PPP in relation to other skin diseases in of 0.37 percent of patients. Patients with signs of psoriasis elsewhere on the body were excluded in this study. The study dates back to 1971 and this percentage is more likely much higher now. Generally there are not many statistics on PPP and there is very little information available.

PPP usually develops in middle-aged adults and seem to be more frequent in women than men. I was 33 when I was diagnosed with PPP. At that time, I was a busy professional with a 3 year old daughter, and becoming sick was not part of my plan

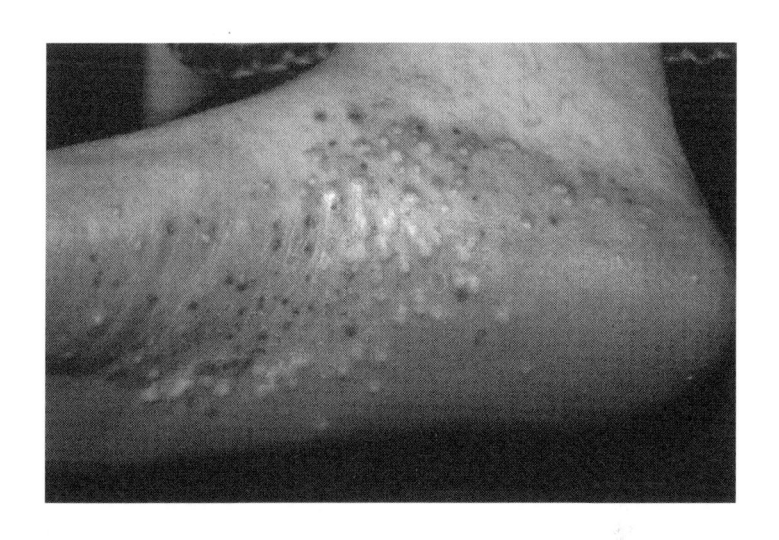

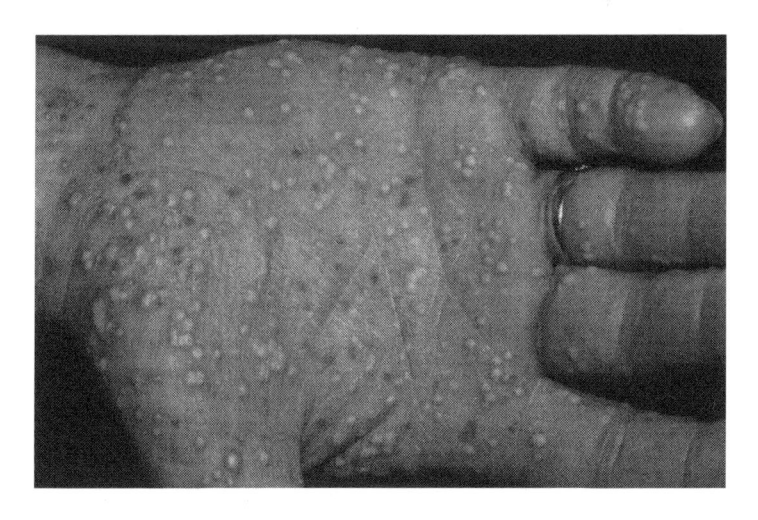

A foot and hand covered in a PPP outbreak. Photo in courtesy of Dr. Gary M. White, MD from ww.regionalderm.com

PPP – WHAT CAN A CASE STUDY TELL US?

I want to describe a recent case study that breaks down possible causal factors for PPP. A Swedish case study from 2005 compared 60 women with PPP against a control group. (Numbers were that 60 women had PPP, compared to the 154 women selected at random.) Significantly, 95% of the women with PPP had been smokers or were currently still smoking. Of the patients (smokers) had no lesions at the time of blood sampling, but had shown typical mild to moderate PPP at earlier examination. Eight of these patients had psoriasis as well, which was usually mild and localized to the extremities.

The study found that smoking plays a major part in the onset of PPP, even though no one is sure why. This study also found that PPP is associated with an increase of calcium in the body and a significant decrease in the PTH levels compared with healthy people who do not suffer from PPP.

The **PTH (Parathyroid hormone)** is secreted by the parathyroid glands and is the most important regulator of calcium levels in the blood and within the bones. The parathyroid glands are small endocrine glands in the neck of humans and other tetrapods that produce parathyroid hormone.

Parathyroid hormone (PTH) allows your body to pull calcium from your bones and tells your body to start making more activated vitamin D to absorb more calcium in the gut. This helps your body keep a narrow and healthy range of calcium in the blood. When calcium is just right in your blood, your PTH will lower and stop pulling calcium from your bones. None of the patients from the Swedish study used calcium and/or vitamin D supplements. The higher calcium levels are thought to be due to the lower PTH levels.

PPP, gluten and other illnesses

Gluten intolerance and sensitivity has a strong connection with PPP. This will be discussed further in the section on leaky gut, but it is remarkable that nearly twenty percent of the patients with PPP had clinical gluten intolerance. Many people in the general population (both with and without PPP) have signs of gluten sensitivity, and may show symptoms of intolerance after significant exposure to gluten, although small amounts may be digested.

In the case study, of the women with PPP, a surprising number, (18%), also had celiac disease (gluten intolerance). The patients with PPP and with gluten intolerance had significantly lower blood calcium levels than the patients with PPP and no evidence of gluten intolerance. Only one of the eleven patients with gluten intolerance had a previously known celiac disease, the other ten were identified after screening for antibodies against gluten, which was performed in all patients with PPP. Those who were found to have antibodies were further examined through a gastroscopy (unpublished data).

Of patients with diabetes, two had Type 1 diabetes since adolescence; however, fifteen patients developed Type 2 diabetes following their diagnosis of PPP. Of those, approximately half required oral anti diabetic medication to control their diabetes, the other followed a dietary regimen to ensure optimal blood glucose levels.

In terms of mental health of the group with PPP, 15 percent had long term depressive symptoms such as clinical depression, anxiety, or insomnia, and one had schizophrenia. Two patients had bipolar disorder. Researchers could not determine whether the link between depression and PPP were due to the general discomfort of PPP and the associated decrease in quality of life, or if there was another factor.

PPP and smoking

Most significantly, in the Swedish study researchers found that smoking plays a major part in the onset of PPP, even though no one is sure why. In a Japanese study (2002) performed on golden hamsters, smoking tobacco was found to have a significant effect on the parathyroid gland. The study found that smoking exposure increases the cellular activity of the parathyroid gland, and stimulates the cell cycle and release of PTH; additionally, smoking exposure promotes bone resorption. Bone resorption is the process by which osteoclasts (a type of bone cell) break down bone and release the minerals, resulting in a transfer of calcium from bone fluid to the blood.

PPP and depleted vitamins and minerals

When there are high levels of calcium in the blood as seen in the patients with PPP, there's an associated decrease in PTH release from the parathyroid gland, that results in fewer total osteoclasts (bone cells) and lower levels of activity, resulting in less overall bone resorption. Bone resorption is stimulated or inhibited by signals from other parts of the body, depending on the demand for calcium.

There is no research as to why this is connected to PPP outbreaks, but a small Danish study revealed a significant decrease in bone mineral density in patients with PPP. The study suggests that PPP patients have a decreased bone mineral density due to primary pathogenic events (pathogenic = infectious agent such as bacteria, fungus parasite which causes disease in the host), and that osteoporosis may be an additional problem for patients with PPP.

In terms of low bone mineral density, the Swedish study did not rule out the possibility of a disturbance in either the function or production of vitamin D in PPP. Known as the 'sunshine vitamin' as sunlight is a major source of vitamin D, vitamin D increases the body's calcium absorption. In the Swedish study there is no mention of vitamin K2 and its supportive role in increasing calcium and phosphate absorption in the intestinal tract. Although vitamin D3 increases mineral absorption, it can't do it without the help of vitamin K2.

Vitamin K2 is necessary to convert a critical bone-building protein called **osteocalcin**. Osteocalcin is a necessary protein that helps maintain calcium homeostasis in bone tissue. It works with osteoblast cells to build healthy bone tissue. Inadequate K2 inhibits osteocalcin production and reduces calcium flow into bone tissue. This leads to reduced bone mass and a weakened bone matrix.

Vitamin D3 and K2 play an essential role in calcium uptake into skeletal bone tissue. Several studies have shown a synergistic effect of vitamin K2 and D3. These studies show that this combination enhanced osteocalcin accumulation in bone cells. This increased osteocalcin formation significantly improves bone mineral density. A recent study of almost 40,000 Dutch men and women found that increased intake of vitamin K2 may reduce the risk of developing type2 diabetes.

A major source of vitamin K2 is your body's own production by the good bacteria in the intestines. Long-term use of antibiotics can cause a vitamin K2 deficiency by killing these crucial bacteria. Sources of vitamin K2 from food include natto (a Japaneses dish of fermented soy beans), hard and soft cheeses, egg yolk, pure or non-processed organic butter, chicken liver, salami, chicken breast, and ground beef.

PPP is complex disease and seems to be triggered by and affected by a combination of factors. One potential factor is the abnormal cell activity in the parathyroid gland from smoking. Additional factors may include the imbalance of the gut flora caused by antibiotics and the disturbance of D3 uptake, as well as the lack of the vitamin K2 which inhibits the body's natural process of calcium distribution.

TODAY'S MEDICAL TREATMENT OF PPP – POTIONS AND LOTIONS

Topical ointment and treatments

There are various conventional treatments for PPP; however most of them are not very effective, and responses to individual treatments are variable and unpredictable -- and if they do work it's often for a shorter period of time. Once PPP is established it may last for decades and impairs the mobility of the hands and feet, causing severe pain, itching and embarrassment.

I was prescribed two different topical medications, and met with no success before I decided to start a more holistic approach. In a study from 2006 by The Cochrane Collaboration, they had gathered and reviewed all available studies about PPP, they concluded that although several treatments improve the symptoms of chronic palmoplantar pustulosis, **no treatment was shown to suppress the condition completely.**

Oral retinoid therapy (acitretin) appears to be helpful at relieving symptoms, particularly if combined with **PUVA** (a combination treatment consisting of **Psoralens (P)**, then exposing the skin to **UVA** (long wave ultraviolet radiation). One drawback is that retinoids are highly teratogenic. (A teratogen disrupts the development of an embryo or fetus and causes birth defects.) Acitret, ciclosporin and tetracycline antibiotics can also provide some relief for PPP symptoms. Topical treatments are generally less helpful, but the efficiency of topical corticosteroids increased by occlusion with hydrocolloid been found to be effective. As yet there is no ideal treatment for chronic palmoplantar pustulosis, though oral retinoids, particularly when combined with **Psoralens** and **ultraviolet radiation (PUVA)**, may help.

Ointments

Topical treatments alone tend to be ineffective for PPP, although some patients may benefit from using emollient creams or ointments, particularly when the disease is mild. These can safely be used as frequently as the patient wishes. PPP is relatively resistant to even the most potent topical treatments; this is likely due in part to the thickness of palmar and plantar skin. Commonly used topical medications for PPP include corticosteroids, vitamin D analogues, keratolytics, anthralin, coal tar, and tazarotene, these stronger type of creams should not be used more than once a day for the maximum of 4 weeks.

Hydrocolloid plasters and gel

A hydrocolloid dressing is a wafer type of dressing that contains gel-forming agents that doesn't adhere to the wound, only to the intact skin around the wound. For me, the hydrocolloid plasters were a lifesaver during my time of illness, they stopped the skin from becoming hard and scaly, and this resulted fewer cracks forming and in less bleeding. With hydrocolloid plasters on I could even do the dishes and take baths as they are water proof.

Coal tar

Some dermatologists advocate the use of tar and coal tar preparations for PPP to be used to help reduce thick scaling. Treatment can be messy, but modern refined tar preparations are less smelly and messy than the traditional unrefined products. Many applications can be purchased over the counter. There is a study by Kumar et al, where 76.5% of patients treated with 6% crude coal tar ointment during the night for 8 weeks showed greater than 50% improvement with no reported side effects.

PUVA

PUVA or photo chemotherapy is a type of ultraviolet radiation treatment (phototherapy) used for severe skin diseases. **PUVA** is a combination treatment which consists of applying **Psoralens (P)** to the affected area, and then exposing the skin to **UVA** (long wave ultraviolet radiation). Psoralen is a natural product which occurs naturally in the seeds of Psoralea corylifolia, as well as in the common fig, celery, parsley, West Indian satinwood, and in all citrus fruits.

Biologics

Some people with PPP have been successful and ended up in remission from their PPP after receiving biologics, but for some their PPP were triggered first after receiving a biologic for other health reasons.

Biologic drugs are given by injection or intravenous (IV) infusion and is a protein-based drug derived from living cells cultured in a laboratory (cells from human or mice etc...). While biologics have been used to treat disease for more than 100 years, modern-day techniques have made biologics much more widely available as treatments, especially in the last decade. Biologics are different from traditional systemic drugs that impact the entire immune system, instead they are set out to target specific parts of the immune system, such as block the action of a specific T cell, or block proteins in the immune system, such as tumor necrosis factor-alpha (TNF-alpha), interleukin 17-A, or interleukins 12 and 23. These cells and proteins all play a major role in developing psoriasis.

According to the-dermatolagist.com, because patients with PPP make up such a small percentage of the total population of psoriasis patients, and the disease is limited and often falls below the 10% inclusion criteria for systemic trials, many more studies are needed in this area.

There have been studies where PPP sufferers had remission from taking a biologic called Efalizumab, but

Efalizumab is no longer available on the market due to an increased risk of progressive multifocal leukoencephalopathy (PML), a rare and usually fatal disease of the central nervous system. Today biologics normally used for psoriasis such as Humira, Enbrel, and Amevive, as these have been shown in many small trials and case reports to also be effective for PPP.

Anyone considering taking a biologic drug should talk with his or her doctor about the short- and long-term side effects and risks. It is important to weigh the risks against the benefits of using the drugs.

PPP AND ME

My Story, My Journey

After many visits to different doctors, I was finally diagnosed with PPP in May 2011 by a dermatologist. I had always been eating healthy and quite health conscious until my daughter was born in July 2008. In 2009 when I went back to work I kept breastfeeding my little girl, and the older she got, the more energy and vitamins she sucked out of me (literally). This resulted in me always being hungry. To still that hunger I would eat anything that was available and convenient, including loads of junk food like pizza, hamburgers, sweets, chocolate, crisps etc... At the same time I was losing weight rapidly and I ended up looking like skin and bones.

To add to this I was working full time and doing tons of overtime in a job that was filled with a lot of negative stress. Working was stressful, and being a mom to a toddler was extremely stressful. Around this time I started to smoke again, I had successfully managed to quit when I got pregnant. I was trying to cope with stress overload in any way I could.

One day during that time I woke up with a severe pain in my heart, my chest ached, it was excruciating. I remember thinking this is not good, I'm going to have to make changes in my diet and I need to slow down, or I'm going to kill myself. But nothing really changed and my work situation grew even worse.

I quit breastfeeding my daughter when she turned 2, but found it hard to change my bad diet due to all the stress in work. I started to gain weight but the food I ate didn't really contain any vitamins and nourishment. I was sick a lot with loads of colds that I wasn't able get rid of. I also developed rosacea in my face and I looked like I've been on an alcohol bender for weeks.

In January 2011 I got an infection in the gums around my wisdom tooth. The pain was horrific, and the dentist gave me antibiotics to get rid of the infection. After that, all my problems really started.

A few weeks after the dentist visit I started to notice perhaps 20 pin-sized red dots under the sole of my left foot. I showed them to my twin sister, who's a nurse but she had no idea of what it was. After a few weeks they started to get really itchy but they remained red and pin-sized.

One morning in March 2011 I woke up with red bumps and blisters all over my feet, hands, bum, thighs and genital area. The itch and pain was so severe I could not walk. I managed somehow to get to the ER (by public transport – imagine that). At the ER they had no idea what this strange rash was. Doctors suggested maybe herpes or the foot and mouth disease. A gynecologist examined me and diagnosed me with scabies. She told me I had to use scabies cream once or twice a day all over my body, apart from my face, and the rest of the family needed to be treated as well.

I was so depressed leaving the hospital. The fact some little insects/parasites were living on my skin made me want to throw up. Putting on the cream, especially on the genital area, was so painful I cried. My little girl screamed out in pain when we covered her in the cream. My husband couldn't bear the pain and got into the shower to wash it off straight away.

I felt like the worst mom ever, and at the same time I couldn't understand where we could have possibly contracted scabies. We hadn't slept in any place other than home, nor been on a holiday abroad recently. There were no other children in my daughter's playgroup who had scabies. Today I know the outbreak I got is called generalized pustular psoriasis.

A few weeks passed and the "scabies" would not go away. All the bumps and blisters around the genital area were gone but they remained on the sole of my right foot and the palm of my left hand. My daughter developed bumps around her genital area and bum, but they were more likely the result of the very strong scabies cream. Around this time I woke up with the worse strep throat infection (tonsillitis) I ever experienced. So another doctor visit was needed. I was prescribed penicillin and home I went. After the two week course of penicillin was over, the strep throat infection came back. I went to the doctor again who this time gave me stronger antibiotics.

This time I also mentioned my hand and foot problems and asked a bunch of questions. Are my skin problems connected with my tonsillitis? I told him I've been treated for scabies and wasn't the scabies supposed to be gone by now? Could my skin problems be something other than scabies?

The doctor didn't really answer my questions, he just said no, it's not connected, and that he had no idea what was on my foot and hand. The doctor shrugged his shoulders and mumbled that it had something to do with my shoes.

It didn't matter that I cried and begged to be sent to a specialist. I was advised to go home and to get some sleep.

The tonsillitis kept coming back, and after the seventh time and my seventh course of antibiotics within a few months I was finally getting a referral and was sent to a dermatologist to have my foot and hand checked out, but more so because the state of my face (rosacea). The doctor also promised to book an appointment with a throat, ear and nose specialist due to all my strep throat infections.

At the dermatologist clinic after telling my story, the kind skin doctor looked at me and said "You've got PPP, and for the record, you have never had scabies."

He explained that a scabies outbreak is more often seen between the fingers and looks very different.

I cried with relief. Finally somebody was taking me seriously. I had an accurate diagnosis. Relief was soon followed by shock and disbelief – I never had scabies?

All those weeks of depression, and all those long hours of doing laundry every day to scrub and kill the scabies parasites, all the times I avoided shaking someone's hand, and going out of my way to prevent any skin to skin contact with people, and hanging my outdoor jacket far away from where everybody else in work were hanging theirs (in case the scabies would crawl over to their clothes), and not the least, all the pain I had put my daughter through, was all for nothing.

All that for nothing. Because a doctor was wrong, and didn't take the time to understand me or my situation. Now in the dermatologist's office, I finally had some answers.

The dermatologist explained **PPP is an autoimmune skin disease** and it's mostly female smokers who contract it, he also said it is chronic and they know it often shows after an infection such as tonsillitis (strep throat infection). He prescribed some very strong cortisone cream (betnovat with chinoform) for my foot and hand, and another cream for my rosacea. It finally looked like things would improve.

After a while my face got a little bit better, but not my foot or my hand. In fact they gradually got worse. (I later noticed that with every PPP outbreak there seemed to be a cycle of three weeks.) The blisters, cracks and patches of dry skin just got bigger and bigger. I went back to the dermatologist and he explained to me that PPP is a very hard to treat and the cream doesn't really work for most people; he then prescribed even stronger cortisone in liquid form (Betnovat with strong steroids) and some plaster to put on my foot (Duoderm).

This treatment actually helped heal the cracks in my foot and hand, and I soon was able to walk normally again without a limp. But it did not stop the PPP outbreaks. The doctor told me there is no point in me going back to him, unless I wanted to try some tablets which basically would suppress my immune system completely. **(The treatment of autoimmune diseases is typically with immunosuppression—medication which decreases the immune response.)**

Immunosuppressants have serious side effects, including increasing your risk of other serious infections. The doctor explained that if I got pregnant within two years after taking the medication, my child would have a very high chance of having birth defects. This didn't really feel like an option to me, even though I wasn't planning any more children.

I mentioned to the dermatologist that I had done some of my own research about the disease and due to its autoimmune nature, it must have something to do with the immune system being completely shut down and there must be away to boost it. I told him about all my strep throat infections.

He replied, "Yes, the immune system is complex, and no ,I can't help you with your strep throat infections; you'll need to see a nose, ear and throat specialist for that." Basically he wasn't interested in hearing my theories about the immune system and it's functioning.

I tried to take matters into my own hands, and thought more medical care could help me. In November 2011 I decided to have my wisdom tooth pulled out, thinking that's how it all started and maybe somehow it was the cause of all my problems. It only made things worse. It cost me a fortune to have it taken out, and I was in severe pain afterwards. To top it off, my PPP worsened to the extent that I got thousands of new blisters on my foot and hundreds on my hand.

At this point I made an appointment to have my tonsils taken out. I thought that if it wasn't the tooth, it was defiantly the tonsils, and the recurring strep throat infections that were causing all these problems for me. I had them taken out in January 2012 and went through ten days of the most severe and unbearable pain ever experienced. Afterward I had another severe PPP outbreak, and I was totally depressed.

My Own Research

Between all my doctor and dentist visits, I tried to find out as much as possible about PPP. I spent hours and days reading medical journals and articles, websites, and Internet forums by other people who suffered with the same chronic disease. I was basically doing anything to find a cure for PPP. But there's not much information out there, and it didn't take me long to realise a dermatologist wouldn't be able to help, apart from reducing the symptoms a little bit by prescribing various lotions and potions. Apparently PPP is the most difficult form of psoriasis to cure, and things started to look very dark.

I read an article that's still circulating the Internet by a Japanese doctor, Dr. Masaru Maebashi. Dr. Maebashi described how it's possible to cure PPP by taking probiotics and biotin. I tried that for a couple of months, but in my case there were no improvements.

I dove into my research and began to learn about what exactly an autoimmune disease is and what it means to the sufferer. There are many different autoimmune diseases such as cancer, Crohn's disease, Multiple Sclerosis, psoriasis, rheumatoid, arthritis, just to mention a few. I learned they are caused by an imbalance in the immune system; this causes the cells in the body that are meant to fight infections in the body to fight themselves instead.

At this point I realized my immune system was completely messed up – I had reoccurring strep throat infections, thrush infections which would not go away despite using the strongest creams on the market for thrush, continuous colds that I just couldn't kick, gum infections, and constant pustules, bleeding and cracking from PPP. It was all caused by a bad diet, stress, and antibiotics. It doesn't take a lot to figure that even if I got rid of my wisdom tooth or my tonsils, the root cause of the problem was still there, hence I still had PPP.

Questions floated around in my mind. I had so few answers. Nobody seemed to know anything about PPP, other than it's chronic, and lasts a lifetime. My big questions —- like was it even possible to restore my immune system back to what it was before I got sick; and was there any chance at all to get well again?

The doctors weren't able to help me, apart from extracting my tooth and tonsils, and only reduced my PPP symptoms. As an added bonus they gave me the misdiagnosis of scabies. I was losing faith in the medical system.

Like so many, I turned to Dr. Google. I searched for 'how to improve the immune system' and was soon overwhelmed by information. Everyone had an opinion, a tidbit of information, or some kind of plan. But one book stood out. I purchased '<u>The Immune System Cure' by Lorna R. Vanderhaeghe and Patrick J.D Bouic.</u> The book said it's possible to cure the immune system in 30 days. This in-depth book described how the complex immune system works, and why so many people in the Western world suffered from the many different diseases that all stemmed from a non-functional immune system.

The big reasons for an epidemic of autoimmune diseases were stress, antibiotic overuse or misuse,

unhealthy and sedentary lifestyles, poor diet, and in many cases, smoking.

Food was a big factor. The book explained that most food we are eating today lack essential vitamins and minerals that are crucial for our well-being. Most of the food we consume has been frozen, highly processed, and is nutrient-poor and filled with environmental toxins. The underlying message in the book is change your diet, stop eating fast food and try to buy as much organic food as possible, and be sure to cook it yourself. Simple advice, but hard to follow in our busy modern lifestyles. Other advice was to cut down on caffeine, alcohol, fizzy drinks, gluten and sugar; and to take vitamin supplements, but most importantly, don't stress.

I found stress being the trickiest part to combat. If you're like me, and have a stressful job combined with a small child, you're going to have a serious think what causes stress in your life and how to break that negative cycle.

I thankfully managed to get my health back on track and I'm confident you are able to do so too.

UNDERSTANDING THE IMMUNE SYSTEM

How does the immune system work?

First of all it's important to explain how the immune system works, for you to get a better understanding of what's happening inside your body when the system is not working as it should, and to understand why you're going to have to make certain life style changes. The immune system is a complex topic, I'll do my best to break it down in a readable and digestible matter.

Cells in general

All the parts of our bodies are made up of cells. There is no such thing as a typical cell as our bodies has many different kinds of cells. Even though they might look different under a microscope, most cells have the same chemical and structural features in common. In the human body there are about 200 different types of cells.

Cells are the fundamental units of life, these are the bricks from which all our tissues and organs are made of; they are also the smallest components considered to be living organisms in our bodies. Your cells are constantly communicating with each other, responding to the environment and to the signals they receive from what we touch and how we move. We need to be kind to these little ones; they are everything that the body is built upon.

All cells have a **membranes**. Cell membranes are the outer layers that hold the cell together. They let the nutrients from what we are eating pass into the cell and waste products pass out. Not everything can pass through a cell membrane. What gets through and what doesn't depends on both the size of the particle trying to get in and the size of the opening in the membrane.

Cells also have a **nucleus.** This is the cell's control center. Cells continually divide to make more cells for growth and repair in our body. The nucleus contains essential information that allows cells to reproduce, or make more cells. Another important part of a cell is the mitochondrion. This is the part of the cell where nutrients and oxygen combine to make energy. If your cells cannot operate efficiently, the functioning of your tissues and organs (that are made of cells) will become compromised, and you can experience diminish physical functioning. This will then trigger a host of health conditions and diseases. By keeping your cells well nourished, you are keeping yourself well nourished.

The Immune Cells

The immune system is a very complex system in our body; acting as a defense mechanism, the immune system attacks foreign invaders that our body doesn't recognize. It's constantly working and searching out and destroying any health damaging agents such as bacteria, viruses, fungi, parasites, cancerous cells, and toxins.

When functioning properly it is very powerful, and the immune system is what keeps us healthy and well.

The immune system is composed of many interconnected cell types that collectively protect the body from invaders. Our body contains two types of blood cells – white and red. The white cells are our defense against invaders, and work as part of the immune system. The white blood cells are born, just like the red blood cells, in the bone marrow of the long bones in our body. These cells are long-lived and carry the memory of past infections. If you happen to be affected by the same virus later, your immune system will remember this invader and immediately respond and start to produce antibodies. You will not even notice you caught it. This is the reason that if you had an illness such as chicken pox, you will not have it again, as the cells will remember this antigen and actively mobilize against it.

There are different types of white cells, called **neutrophils (polymorphs), lymphocytes, eosinophils, monocytes, and basophils**. They travel in the bloodstream and react to different types of infection caused by bacteria, viruses, or other pathogens. Neutrophils engulf bacteria and destroy them by using special chemicals. Eosinophils and monocytes also work by swallowing up foreign particles in the body.

Basophils are capable of ingesting foreign particles and produce heparin and histamine (chemicals which induce inflammation), and are often associated with responding to parasites, asthma and allergies and contribute to the severity of these reactions such as itchiness, swelling of the tongue, vomiting, diarrhea, hives often caused by cow's milk, peanuts, eggs, shellfish, tree nuts, rice, and fruit.

Inflammation is part of your body's natural immune response. Damage to your tissues causes the release of chemicals into the blood. These chemicals make blood vessels leaky, helping specialized white blood cells get to where they are needed. They also attract neutrophils and monocytes to the site of the injury, which helps to prevent a bacterial infection from developing.

The **white blood cells** known as **lymphocytes** will develop as they mature in to B-cells where some of them move on from the bone marrow and spread throughout the body via the bloodstream, on to the lymph. The lymph is a fluid that looks a bit like milk and has a similar composition to that of blood plasma. Humans have approximately 500–600 lymph nodes distributed throughout the body, with clusters found in the underarms, groin, neck, chest, and abdomen. After that passage, the cells go on to the thymus gland where they become T-Cells. The thymus is a specialized organ of the immune system, located in front of the heart and behind the breastbone.

Within the **thymus** gland each T-cell is taught how to recognize both good and bad antigens. With the bad ones, I'm referring to the invading antigens and with the good ones I'm referring to the cells we already have in our bodies. In our body we have millions of antigens and each individual T-cell can only learn to recognize one specific antigen. The T-cells and the B-cells need each other to be able to do their job. When there is a foreign antigen in the body, the T-cell tells the B-cell to start producing antibodies, these antibodies are then released in to the blood stream to attack the foreign antigen.

The immune cells are also found in a variety of other organs and tissues, this includes the thymus, bone marrow, tonsils, and lymph nodes, as well as the spleen, appendix, and in the small intestine. The role of the gut in the immune system is a recent topic and new area of understanding the unsung hero of our digestive system.

Interleukins

It is also important to mention **interleukins**, this is a secretion (called cytokine) produced by the immune cells. This secretion works as a biochemical messenger and has many different effects on the immune cells. Researchers continuously discover new ones and there are approximately 30 different types, I will only describe four of them.

Interlerukin-1

This cytokine is involved in the process that induces fever when you are sick. This is very important as fever helps kill or slow down a virus or bacteria.

Interleukin-2

IL-2 helps the different T-cells to destroy an invader. It is very effective in enhancing immune responses against tumors.

Interleukin-4

IL-4 helps the B-cells make antibodies. An overproduction of IL-4 causes allergic responses.

Interleukin-6

IL-6 also helps the B-cells produce antibodies. An abnormal production of IL-6 is associated with autoimmune disease, inflammation, and allergic conditions. Studies show that psoriasis is associated with the T-cells releasing too much of the IL-6 secrete, which increases the production of skin cells.

Normally when the immune system works well it only attacks substances and micro-organism that are considered foreigners to the body, such as bad bacteria or viruses from outside the body like the common cold, or cancer cells inside the body. Unfortunately, sometimes the immune system becomes confused and attacks healthy body cells –basically this is the immune system starting a civil war inside the body which leads to autoimmune diseases.

Autoimmune diseases happen in response to an overproduction of lymphokines by the lymphocites (the white and the B-cells). The lymphokines are a protein that typically delivers information to other immune cells, relaying information telling them what to do. The lyphokines cling on to the other cells and tell them to grow, activate in the case of an infection, eliminate parasites, viruses, and fungi or to destroy other cells. When there's an overproduction of the lymphokines, they promote the B-cells to make antibodies, those antibodies then attack the body and end up creating an autoimmune response.

Immune system nutrition

Cells, tiny building blocks, not only make up every single part of the human body, but they protect it too. The immune system is powerful defender in the war against infection. For cells in the immune system to thrive and function properly, and to avoid illness and autoimmune diseases, you need to nourish these cells by supplying your body with essential vitamins and minerals.

Food is vital, not just to stop your belly from growling, but to give every cell in your body the nutrients they need to grow and function. The only way to do this is to eat healthy and remove the 'bad stuff' from your diet — highly processed food or empty calories that causes inflammation and doesn't have any nutritional value.

You'll also need to reduce stress and start to exercise if that's not already part of your daily regimen. (More about this later in the book.)

But there's a bigger and more central picture to the immune system, and you need look no further than your belly. That's right, your gut. Or rather, your intestinal tract and the flora that reside there. Not many people know but the gut is your biggest immune center. With imbalanced gut flora (too many bad bugs, and not enough good ones), it's just a matter of time before disease enters your life.

Gut flora – what's going on inside us?

As most of us with an autoimmune disease you're probably thinking "Why is my immune system attacking its own army of defenders?" "What can I do to stop this madness?" These were my thoughts after I received my PPP diagnosis. I had a huge drive to understand what was going on inside my body and why.

There are many factors to consider when examining why we end up with a non-functional immune system. The most important factor is the state of our gut (gastrointestinal tract). Scientist has just recently figured out the importance of our gut plays in our overall wellbeing.

Let's begin with a basic overview of the digestion system

The gut is our biggest organ, and spans the length of our body. The mouth is the first part; when we eat, food passes down the **esophagus** (food tube), into the stomach, and then into the small intestine. The small intestine has three sections - the duodenum, jejunum and ileum. The **duodenum** is the first part of the small intestine and extends from the stomach. The duodenum curls around the pancreas creating a c-shaped tube. The **jejunum and ileum** make up the rest of the small intestine and are found coiled in the center of the abdomen. The small intestine is where food is digested and absorbed into the bloodstream.

The first part of the large intestine, called the **caecum**, extends from the ileum. Attached to the caecum is the **appendix**. The large intestine continues upwards from here and is known as the **ascending colon**. The next part of the gut is called the **transverse colon** because it crosses the body. It then becomes the **descending colon** as it heads downwards. The **sigmoid colon** is the s-shaped final part of the colon which leads on to the rectum. Faeces is stored in the rectum and pushed out through the anus when you go to the toilet. The anus is a muscular opening that is usually closed unless you are passing stool. The large intestine absorbs water, and contains food that has not been digested, such as fiber.

But the idea that the only purpose for our gastrointestinal tracts is to digest food is a bit old fashioned.

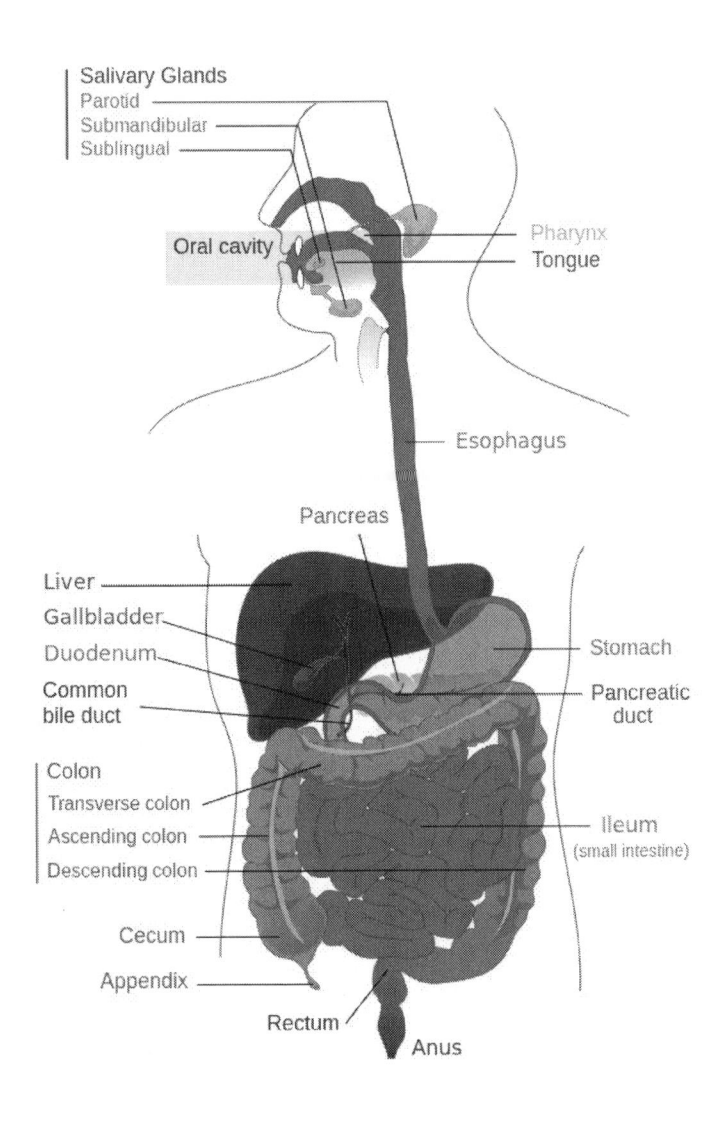

THE GUT AND ITS INHABITANTS

The gut – an essential part of the immune system

A large component of our immune cells and hormone producing cells are located in the intestines. The fact is the gut is the body's largest hormone-producing organ, releasing more than 20 different hormones. Gut hormones are secreted into the blood where they affect function of other parts of the body. Examples of these hormones are ghrelin and leptin which function is to tell the brain when we are hungry and when we are satiated, others are peptide and cholecystokinin which are slowing down the passage of food along the gut, which increases the efficiency of digestion and nutrient absorption after meals, as well as slowing down the emptying of the stomach.

Gut flora microbiome

There are trillions of different bacteria living in our gut. There are ten times more bacteria in our gut compared to our total number of body cells. These gut bacteria represent two kilos of our body weight. These complex colonies of microorganisms serve a vital purpose in stimulating the body's immune system, especially immunoglobulin A (Sec IgA), and representing the first line of immune defense. Sec IgA accounts for approximately 80% of our total immunity, keeping us healthy by suppressing or warding off bacterial, fungal, parasitic and viral pathogens (germs) and toxins, and preventing them from spreading or penetrating through the gut wall to cause infection or disease.

These **microbes** also have over a hundred more genes compared to the human body cell's DNA. Our bodies are quite simply a host environment for bacteria. They use us for their own purposes and only care for their own wellbeing. The molecules produced by the DNA of these bacteria have significant impact on our health. The gut flora determines the quality of the immune system and how much of the available vitamins and minerals the cells will absorb.

Our microbiome, has been linked to everything from obesity to autism, cancer to autoimmune and allergic disorders, and even heart disease and diabetes. Our hectic lifestyle and highly processed, high-carbohydrate and sugar laden diet, as well as the overuse of antibiotics has changed the population of bacteria living in our guts. We are making ourselves sick.

Gut flora also communicate with cells in the immune system, directing the defenders to the microbes that should be attacked, and notifying the immune system of which ones to ignore. In the intestines you will also find a large nervous system with as nerve cells as found in the spinal cord.

The **central vagus nerve** spans from the intestine to all the way up to the brain. The nerve is one of the largest nerve systems in the body, and besides giving output to different organs, the vagus nerve comprises between

80% and 90% of afferent nerves, mostly conveying sensory information about the state of the body's organs to the central nervous system. Current research has found a strong effect gut flora has on our general mood and functioning of the brain.

The problem is most people never think about what happens with whatever they put in their mouth and ends up in their tummy. It doesn't matter if it's food, alcohol, drugs, or vitamins. The fact is everything we digest has to go through an extensive metabolic process. Everything gets broken down to tiny components, and is integrated with hormones, bacteria and cells on a molecular level.

The gut is a dynamic system, all components affect each other and nothing goes by unnoticed. Only now do we understand the microbiome of the gut and its implications for influencing disease. The types of bugs we grow in our intestine determine whether we'll be fat or thin, inflamed or healthy. We're only just beginning to understand that what happens in the gut affects the rest of the body. By changing our diets and the use of pre- and probiotics we can make sure we have a healthy gut environment where the good bacteria can flourish.

We are only as healthy as our gut bacteria. As the father of medicine, Hippocrates, said "Let food be thy medicine and medicine be thy food."

The medical history of bacteria

Scientists and researchers are only in the beginning stages of understanding the importance of the bacteria that reside in and on our bodies. They now look at it as an ecosystem which works very well together. Until recently, the general view has been that most bacteria colonising the human body are bad for us and should be exterminated. Now we know the opposite is true.

Gut flora – why are they it so important?

The role of gut flora is to break down fibre, and gather energy from the fermentation of undigested carbohydrates (sugar) and the subsequent absorption of short-chain fatty acids. They also stimulate cell growth, repress the growth of harmful microorganisms, teach the immune system to respond only to pathogens, and defend against some diseases. The gut flora play an important role in synthesizing biotin, vitamin K2 and D3, as well as metabolizing bile acids, sterols (found naturally in animals, vegetables and cholesterol to name a few) and foreign substances that are not expected to be present such as antibiotics and other chemicals.

The good bacteria in the gut also helps reduce, and in some cases, eliminate, **antinutrients**. One antinutrients is **phytic acid**, which you'll find in seeds, legumes and nuts. The phytic acid binds and prevents the absorption of important minerals that are crucial for us to function properly. If your gut flora are not healthy, diets rich in phytic acid can result in malnutrition. It might be a good idea to exclude antinutrients from your diet until you are healed. When the microbiomes in the gut are fueled with balanced nutrition they are able to create all the vitamins that a human needs.

We are all born without any bacteria in our gut. When a baby is born, its immunity is acquired initially from its mother, first when descending through the birth canal and second, via colostrum and Secretory IgA from breast feeding. The bacteria present in the babies gut supports the development of its immune system, and if challenged by unhealthy foods, toxins, and pathogenic bacteria, the immune system may be over–stimulated. This is now believed to play a huge role in developing disease.

An unbalanced gut flora

Human health, digestion, immune function and metabolic balance depend to such an extent upon maintaining colonies of good bacteria, that some people consider the gut flora to constitute an organ in its own right. An imbalance in the gut flora, leading to the overgrowth of harmful bacteria and yeast in the gut is known as **dysbiosis**. Dysbiosis is believed to be an underlying cause of many serious health complaints such as irritable bowel syndrome (IBS), chronic fatigue, eczema, multiple sclerosis, rheumatoid arthritis and depression. Levels of beneficial bacteria can be adversely affected by a number of factors including disease, the effects of stress, poor diet and the use of antibiotics.

Antibiotic use can deplete entire gut flora colonies, wiping out large numbers of good bacteria and thereby reducing the gut's defenses against illness, inflammation and infection. In the absence of beneficial bacteria, resistant bacteria, parasites, viruses and yeasts are allowed to "over-colonize" the intestinal wall. Intestinal imbalance is now seen to be the main reason behind why the body suddenly becomes sensitive to a particular type of food.

Potential triggers for gut flora disruption include:

- NSAIDs (Non-steroidal anti-inflammatory drugs)

- Immune system dysfunction with low sec IgA production

- Medication such as antibiotics or the birth control pill

- Food toxins mostly from grains and legumes

- Excess carbohydrate, sugar and fructose consumption

- Inflammation from excess total polyunsaturated and omega-6 fat consumption

- Physical conditions such as infections, chronic stress, and lack of sleep

- Improper nutrient intake and deficiency in some critical vitamins and minerals

- Weak immune system (often caused by all of the above)

Gut functioning is affected by the food consumed, physiological stress, the efficiency of your immune system, and the balance of gut flora. If you have specific questions or concerns, please seek professional medical care.

ANTIBIOTICS

Antibiotics are a family of medications used to treat bacterial infections, they will not kill viruses. But just as **probiotics (pro= for; bios = life) support life**, **antibiotics (anti = against; bios = life) are designed to kill**. A course of antibiotics can kill not only harmful bacteria in your gut, but also all the good bacteria, leaving you even more vulnerable to illness.

When antibiotics were discovered approximately 80 years ago, they were seen as a huge medical breakthrough for human health. Antibiotics saved countless lives and have significantly lengthened our lifespans. But that benefit has come with a cost, and it's one that we're only just beginning to understand the full implications of.

We are creating 'super-bugs.' **Antibiotic resistance** occurs when an antibiotic has lost its ability to effectively control or kill bacterial growth. The bacteria are "resistant" to use of a particular antibiotic at the standard dose. We are only now beginning to understand the serious implications of this, as it becomes harder to treat diseases that used to be treated with antibiotics.

The use of antibiotics can impair the gut flora's ability to self-regulate by suppressing bad bacteria and may lead to a range of secondary infections. Two of the most common infections include Clostridium difficile (aka "C-Diff") and Candida albicans (aka "yeast infection") both of which are normally suppressed by secretory Immunoglobulin A and the natural dominance of good bacteria in the gut.

Antibiotic resistance was a problem even when penicillin was being developed. The fact is the first resistant bacterial strains were discovered before the drug was even available to the public. Alexander Fleming who accidentally discovered the drug warned about the risks of antibiotic resistance in his Nobel Prize acceptance speech. Despite these warnings, antibiotics are widely used in both the medical system and the meat industry. Today's food technology makes it difficult to avoid getting second-hand exposure to antibiotics by eating meat from animals that had been treated with antibiotics.

Despite the risk of antibiotic resistance and the long term negative effects on health, the health care system still depends on antibiotic use for treatment of infection. Antibiotics are commonly used in surgery, for transplants and cancer treatments where there is a high risk of infection; as well as to treat more common illnesses such as strep throat, pneumonia, and ear infections. Widespread antibiotic use has become a way of life.

When used properly, antibiotics are effective at killing the harmful bacteria that cause illness and infection. Unfortunately many of the good bacteria inhabiting our bodies are also killed off during these treatments, particularly those in the gut. Normally the good bacteria keep the bad ones in check, but a single course of antibiotics can disrupt the intestinal flora for months afterwards. When the normal intestinal flora are disturbed, the bad bacteria that normally inhabit our gut are th12en free to take over, multiplying unchecked.

Many of us, including me, were given antibiotics frequently as children (to treat ear, kidney and throat infections) or as young adults for skin problems. When antibiotics are used often there is an increased risk of developing more resistant bacterial strains, as a few scattered bacteria initially survive antibiotic treatment then reproduce. Humans may then infect each other with these 'super bugs'.

Antibiotics, especially broad spectrum antibiotics (that kill a large number of bacteria indiscriminately), are the main cause of an unbalanced gut flora. Unfortunately, broad spectrum antibiotics tend to be used more frequently, and wage a war against normal gut flora. Despite the risk of antibiotic resistance and the long term negative effects on health, the health care system is still dependent on using antibiotics for widespread treatment of infection and illness.

Normally the good bacteria keep the bad ones in in check, but a single course of antibiotics can disrupt the intestinal flora for several months afterwards. When the normal intestinal flora is disturbed, the bad bacteria inhabiting our gut may reproduce rapidly, changing the balance of our gut, and affecting our immune system.

One of these bacteria is streptococcus, the agent behind the notorious 'strep throat.' Streptococcus naturally inhabits human skin and the throat, and is the cause of a number of infectious and noninfectious illness such as sepsis, abscesses, respiratory infections, and meningitis. It ranks among the top ten infectious pathogens, affecting 700 million individuals and causing over 500,000 deaths 1`per year globally. Even if potentially harmful bacteria do not cause serious infection, they can go on to create biofilms in the body. Biofilms and the waste products produced by these bacteria are a major cause of inflammation.

Avoiding antibiotics is the best thing you can do to ensure good gut bacteria balance. **Taking quality daily probiotics supplement during a course of antibiotics is a must**. I wish my doctor would have informed me of that when he kept treating me with the same type of antibiotic during my repetitive strep throat infections. Natural sources of probiotics are yogurt, kefir, kimchi, and tempeh, to name a few.

One clinical trial, following 155 hospital patients, found that daily supplementation with a mixture of Lactobacillus acidophilus, Bifidobacterium bifidum,Lactobacillus acidophilus and Bifidobacterium animalis (var lactis) alongside antibiotic treatment significantly reduced the number of antibiotic resistant strains by more than 70% compared to those taking a placebo.

Taking probiotics alongside a course of antibiotics has been shown to help prevent some of the problems caused by antibiotic overuse. It can also help support efficient functioning of the immune system, help keep the intestinal barrier (that layer of mucous and good bacteria that helps support proper immune function) healthy, and help your normal intestinal flora to recover more quickly. Probiotics should be a part of your daily diet if you have disrupted gut flora.

BACTERIAL BIOFILMS

What causes biofilm and what harm can it do?

I have already mentioned that the bacteria in your gut creates **biofilms**, I want to go a bit deeper what type of harm these biofilms can cause if not removed. Opportunists of the bacteria world, biofilms develop almost anywhere long as there are microorganisms, moisture, nutrients, and a suitable surface. They are found in fresh and salt water, in the desert, inside oil pipelines and inside the human body. Biofilms can stick to almost any surface such as medical equipment, countertops, and human tissue.

In a healthy gut that is filled with beneficial microflora, the biofilm that they create is thin mucus. This healthy biofilm allows the passage of nutrients through the intestinal wall. Healthy gut biofilm is lubricating and anti-inflammatory. In a healthy gut flora the biofilms release vitamins that are taken up by intestinal cells to provide the needs of the body. People on a healthy diet with a normal gut flora, can subsist on very limited diets without vitamin deficiency diseases, because all of the vitamins can be obtained from bacteria growing in films coating the lining of the gut.

But the problem is when the bad bacteria in an unbalanced gut flora creates biofilm formations. One common type of biofilm is the dental plaque that causes cavities and gum disease. In the 1990s the concept of biofilm was introduced to the medical community. Doctors began to see the connection between chronic, low-grade infections and the growth of biofilms.

Dental professionals found biofilms in plaque on teeth. Internal cases of chronic infection inside the body caused by biofilms have taken longer to prove, but testing has shown that many troublesome diseases are caused by microbial populations at their core. Peptic ulcers, once thought to be caused by stress, have been proved to be caused by bacterial communities of H.pylori which is a bacteria estimated nearly half of the population carries, although not everyone show any symptoms. The cyclical flare-up of children's recurrent earaches is an example of a typical biofilm-based infection.

Biofilms are created as a result of a mechanism for protecting against environmental attack. In a biofilm a colony of bacteria creates a slime (called matrix) that they surround themselves with. You can compare it to an egg, where the egg yolk is the bacteria colony and the egg white is the biofilm.

When bad bacteria develop biofilms they create the ultimate defense mechanism. In their biofilms they thrive and multiply, and are protected from our own immune system. The slime is built on a 'metal and mucus structure' that acts as an impenetrable shield, making it difficult or even impossible to attack the residing intruders with antibiotics or probiotics alone. The bacteria inside a biofilm are able to communicate with each other and exchange signaling molecules important in biofilm formation.

The bad news is an **unhealthy gut biofilm**, created by the bad bacteria, reduces nutrient absorption, which results in our immune cells are not getting all the nutrients they need to function properly. These biofilms also cause inflammation, and store toxins like heavy metals. This means as long as the biofilms exist in your body, it doesn't matter if you take vitamin supplements, your body will not absorb most of them anyway. In my case, I started to lose my hair due to zinc deficiency. My doctor diagnosed zinc deficiency base on clinical signs – my nails were covered in white dots and my dry, brittle hair that was falling out. I started to take zinc supplements as the doctor advised, but unfortunately without any benefit.

The strong shield-like protection that biofilm provides bad bacteria is one reason why some infections are so difficult to treat. Yeasts, parasites, and bacteria find shelter in the biofilm matrix, evading an onslaught of even the strongest of medications.

Infections related to bad bacteria biofilms include

- Chronic fatigue syndrome and fibromyalgia, which are often thought to have an infectious root.

- Systemic Candida overgrowth.

- Heartburn or GERD (gastroesophageal reflux).

- Small intestine bacterial overgrowth (SIBO), which includes symptoms like heartburn, bloating, gas, abdominal cramping, brain fog, arthritis, acne, and other skin conditions such as psoriasis and rosacea.

- Irritable bowel syndrome, ulcerative colitis, and Crohn's disease.

- Unhealthy biofilm allows some infections to carry on for years. This means that the body may become more prone to other autoimmune diseases, as well as other chronic degenerative diseases.

I'm not saying everyone who suffers from PPP has biofilms, but it is quite possible you may have biofilm if you have used antibiotics repeatedly. This is even more likely given that strep throat infections are a major trigger for the onset of PPP.

Part of treating PPP then becomes ensuring your gut flora is healthy. Doing so will reduce inflammation, as well as enhance the absorption of nutrients such as biotin, D3 and K2. The only way to tackle the inflammation caused by biofilm is to breakdown and destroy their matrix. Ways to do this naturally include doses of colloidal Silver or Apple Cider Vinegar. Colostrum has also being shown to be successful breaking down both biofilms and the creation of them.

YEAST INFECTIONS

Just like the bad bacteria in your gut, you naturally find yeast in your body. If everything is functioning normally they do not cause any harm, the most common fungus or yeast using us as their host is **candida**. Candida is a yeast fungus that is part of our normal gut flora. It's normally located in the mouth, vagina, and the intestinal tract. There are more than 80 different types of candida, and candida albicans is the most common one.

Normally the immune system and the good **bacteria lactobacillus** keep yeast in balance, but with an impaired immune system yeast can become so numerous they cause infection. The candida fungus is opportunistic and aggressive, if it has an opportunity to grow and take over an environment, it will. In low levels, it is not harmful to the body, and candida itself is a source of food for beneficial gut flora that help fight infectious disease. As long as the amount of yeast in the body remains small, internal balance is maintained and all is well. The harm is when there is an overgrowth of candida – that's when the troubles begins.

Yeast overgrowth can be triggered by a number of things.

- A diet high in sugar

- An imbalanced immune system

- Stress

- Bacterial overgrowth in the gut

- Oral contraceptive use or an imbalance in estrogen

Candida grow in a moist and warm environment, about 37 degrees or the average human body temperature. At least 25% of the population is estimated to have excess candida in Western populations. Candida can develop into a fungal disease (**mycoses**) and create major problems in the body. Candida may then invade all the organs of the body; but it thrives especially well in the digestive tract and the intestines. If candida enters the blood stream it can be fatal.

The body uses glucose (sugar) as its primary fuel to create energy; however, glucose is the primary nutrient that fuels candida growth. When candida absorbs glucose, it triggers a fermentation process that creates two by-products – alcohol and acetaldehyde. Both alcohol and acetaldehyde are absorbed into the bloodstream and affect the brain the same way that a few glasses of alcohol would. This creates a feeling of intoxication, also known as 'brain fog,' resulting in reduced concentration, reduced productivity and impaired mental clarity. Acetaldehyde can cause feelings of nausea and is the substance that is responsible for the classic symptoms of a hangover.

Candida symptoms

The symptoms of candida overgrowth in women include a rash or vaginal yeast infections. Other symptoms may include bloating, excessive gas, fatigue, dizziness, weight gain, food allergies, excessive mucus production, extreme cravings for sweet food, problems with the skin and scalp, bad breath, and night sweats. When candida affect the thymus it disrupts production of T cells, thereby affecting the immune system's ability to respond to alien invaders and illness.

In the book **Magstarkt** by Martina Johansson, a Swedish engineer in biochemistry and biophysics, she explains that just as antibiotics can reduce the presence of healthy intestinal bacteria, the hormone system may be triggered to change the PH balance of the stomach. If the pH rises the stomach will become too alkaline, leading to a less welcoming environment for the good bacteria that live there. When the good bacteria die, more opportunistic organisms that thrive an alkaline environment will take over, and candida is one of them.

In consuming several courses of antibiotics, birth control pills, and a high intake of carbohydrates and sugars, the candida population can explode, taking over the intestinal tract and other parts of the body, while driving out good bacteria. Candida also interfere with digestion and the absorption of nutrients. Candida bind to hormones, thereby changing their shape so that they no longer fit in to their original receptors. This means that certain hormones may be 'deactivated' as they can no longer trigger change and communication through hormone receptors, leading to potential hormonal imbalance.

Martina Johansson also explains that residues from candida produce false estrogen; this tricks the body into thinking that it has produced sufficient quantities of estrogen and it gives signals to the body indicating that now it's time to cease production. Similar signals can also be sent to the thyroid gland which than reduces the production of the thyroid hormone. When estrogen or thyroid hormones are low, your metabolism slows and you start to feel cold and tired. The thyroid gland and the adrenal gland activity also indirectly control gastric acid production in the stomach. When these glands do not work effectively, gastric acid concentration will also become lower. All this will eventually lead to reduced nutrient absorption, especially B vitamins, folic acid, vitamin K2, and iron.

When gastric acid is too low, the stomach doesn't always close the **cardia** tight enough (the opening into the stomach); allowing gastric acid to seep out, and triggering acid reflux or heartburn. This may be diagnosed as too much stomach acid, but it is actually a symptom of the opposite. Acid reflux is usually treated with drugs that neutralize the gastric acid, which eliminate the symptoms but results in reduced secretion of digestive enzymes. This means that the food is both too acidic and less finely divided when it enters the digestive tract.

Candida grows very long roots called rhizoids that can puncture the mucosal lining of the intestine. When the mucosal lining becomes damaged, we develop a condition called **leaky gut syndrome**. This means that the mucosal lining of the digestive tract has holes in it, allowing candida to pass through it into the bloodstream.

Due to the correlation with estrogen, problems with candida over-growth almost exclusively affect women. It negatively affects fertility and may lead to hormonal imbalances, this in turn affects metabolism and intestinal movement. When this happens constipation and high blood sugar tend to be the result, which leads to weight gain or difficulty in losing weight.

Because the intestines, estrogen, and the thyroid gland are connected to problems associated with candida over-growth, they can be resolved by restoring the intestinal gut flora to heal the gut. There are many anecdotal stories from PPP sufferers who cured themselves from PPP by going on a 'Candida diet' (a diet that excludes carbs and sugar in any form apart from natural sugars in fruit and vegetables). Candida may also be a reason why PPP mostly affects women.

If you suspect you have Candida, it is also important to bear in mind that candida can also produce biofilms the same way as bacteria does. To successfully remove candida, their biofilms need to be destroyed. I will explain how to do this in the chapter on how to repair a broken immune system.

GLUTEN

Our understanding about the negative health effects related to gluten has increased dramatically over the past few years; although best known for affecting those with celiac disease, gluten can negatively affect many others as well.

Gluten (from Latin gluten "glue") is a protein composite found in wheat and other related grains, including barley and rye. Gluten gives elasticity to bread dough, helping it rise and keep its size and is also what gives the final product a chewy texture. Gluten, especially wheat gluten, is also the basis used for imitation meats (such as faux beef, chicken, and pork). When cooked in broth, gluten absorbs some of the surrounding liquid and flavor, and becomes firm to the bite.

Today's wheat has been significantly refined and is distinct from the wheat we used in the past. There is 10 times more gluten in the wheat we use today, compared to the amount 50 years ago. When it comes to specific foods that humans have not adapted to digest, wheat and gluten protein are probably at the top of that list. Unfortunately wheat is omnipresent in our society today – from soy sauce to nearly all commercially baked goods, and many surprise appearances in processed foods. It's practically inescapable.

Unfortunately, many health conditions are related to our high consumption of wheat. There are many reports of positive changes to one's health that are noticed after removing wheat and other gluten-containing grains from the diet for a period of at least three months.

More and more of my fellow Swedes, including children and adults, suffer from gluten intolerance. Only a third of those who are sick are being diagnosed. The problem is symptoms can be vague, such as fatigue, upset stomach, rashes and difficulty conceiving. It has long been known that there is a link between gluten intolerance and several other autoimmune diseases. Previously this has been explained as there may be a common genetic factor being triggered, but recent research shows that gluten itself may be the common denominator.

Nearly one million people in Sweden (approximately one in ten) have an autoimmune disease. The most common include rheumatoid arthritis (RA), multiple sclerosis, celiac disease (gluten intolerance), alopecia, Type 1 diabetes, hyperthyroidism, autoimmune thyroiditis, vitiligo, Crohn's, ulcerative colitis and IBS (not currently recognized as autoimmune). At one in ten people suffering from an autoimmune disease, the healthcare costs are astronomical.

As mention earlier, autoimmune diseases attack the body's own tissue, causing different symptoms depending on the type of tissues are attacked. The reasons for autoimmune diseases are both hereditary and environmental. Those who have an autoimmune disease have a genetic predisposition that is triggered by one or more environmental factors, and gluten may be one of those factors. But because the vast and overwhelming range of diseases related to gluten, doctors often wind up treating the symptoms of gluten intolerance rather than the underlying cause.

Researchers have different views as to whether there is a connection between gluten intolerance and psoriasis. There are several studies indicating that some people with psoriasis have a sensitivity to gluten, and also indicated a correlation between gluten intolerance and PPP. This makes sense as both psoriasis and PPP are autoimmune diseases. Based on these studies and the correlation between PPP and gluten sensitivity, it is worthwhile trying a gluten-free diet for an extended period of time.

LEAKY GUT SYNDROME

Candida and gluten allergies are two problems that are commonly seen together, and both may cause leaky gut syndrome Leaky gut syndrome describes a condition in which the intestinal lining has become more porous (**hyperpermeable**).

Although normally porous, in leaky gut syndrome, the lining develops more holes that are larger in size, thereby the intestines are no longer able to screen out the products that normally do not enter your bloodstream. This results in larger, undigested food molecules and other 'bad stuff' (yeast, toxins, and all other forms of waste) to flow freely into your bloodstream.

A study by researcher Alessio Fasano found that wheat gluten may cause the intestine to leak, even in typically healthy individuals. Previously this phenomenon was known to happen in people who were gluten intolerant and of have Celiac disease, but now it has been discovered that it applies to most people.

Wheat and some other type of grains consist of different types of proteins called gluten. The word "gluten" is an umbrella term for the proteins found inside many grains and seeds, such as wheat, rye, barley, spelt, kamut and triticale.

Leaky gut occurs when the bonds between the cells inside the intestine begin to pass through undigested food protein (macromolecules). The only foods in the blood stream should have been thoroughly broken down components of vitamins, minerals, amino acids, and fatty acids. According to Dr. Fasano, the intestines leak and food protein that is not totally digested ends up in the bloodstream, the immune system will start to attack these foreign particles. This in turn results in inflammation, potentially leading to food sensitivities and autoimmune diseases.

Cycle of inflammation

When the intestines leak, the immune system mistakes non-digested protein for a foreign invader, and attacks. The immune system may also attack the body's own tissue such as the thyroid, liver, or brain. It is therefore critical to stop supplying gluten to the body as may cause hyper permeable intestines and overstimulate the immune system. At the same time it's important to stop the inflammation caused by the leaking gut, as the inflammation starts a domino effect of oxidative stress, which damages the cells in the body.

Fortunately, new cells grow in the intestine within 3-7 days; the intestine can heal very quickly provided that no additional gluten is digested and that there are enough building blocks to repair the damage. It takes very little gluten to cause damage to the intestinal wall, and quantities as little as 1 mg of gluten prevents the intestine from healing. Each time gluten enters the intestine new holes occurs in the intestinal wall, perpetuating the entire cycle.

You need to completely avoid gluten in order to heal the gut. If you eat gluten, the immune system will react and start to make antibodies. These antibodies will remain in the bloodstream up to 3-6 months after you last ate gluten. If you suffer from an autoimmune disease, the immune system will continue to attack its own tissue for up to six months after you stop eating gluten. This is the reason why you are not able to eat gluten 'every once in a while', as the immune system is still overstimulated long after you last ate gluten. To see the beneficial effects of quitting gluten, it needs to be completely eliminated.

All the effects that gluten have on our health are not fully known, but what we do know is that autoimmune diseases are increasing in the Western world. The good news is that both celiac disease and non-celiac gluten intolerance are 100 percent curable. Remove the gluten and the body heals itself.

SIGNS AND SYMPTOMS OF LEAKY GUT

Leaky gut affects your body to different degrees depending on the length of time your intestinal tract has been damaged. The longer the duration of damage, the more severe the resulting ailments.

Early symptoms of leaky gut include:

- flatulence, belching, abdominal pain and bloating
- diarrhea or constipation
- hay fever or other allergies (STB2)

- **Later symptoms of leaky gut include:**

- food allergies and symptoms of IBS
- recurrent infections, chronic fatigue
- gum disease, headaches, migraines, and joint pain
- depression, difficulty concentrating and sleeping, memory difficulties, symptoms of ADD/ADHD
- asthma, eczema, and autoimmune response such as psoriasis, PPP etc.

Symptoms of leaky gut after an extended period of time include illnesses that affect many different parts of the body, such as:

- Gastro-illnesses such as celiac disease, IBD, colitis, Crohn's disease or chronic parasitic infection
- Neuromuscular diseases such as arthritis, MS, Hashimoto's disease, and chronic muscle pain disorders
- Respiratory illnesses such as severe asthma, or ailments related to calcium deficiency such as osteoporosis

Other causes of leaky gut

Wheat and gluten might not be the only causes for leaky gut syndrome. Other causes may include:

Other foods such as pasteurized milk, processed foods, soy sauce, sugar, bad fats, or excessive salt and alcohol.

Dysbiosis, this is an imbalance in the intestinal flora with too few good intestinal bacteria and an overgrowth of negative ones.

Environmental toxins including household chemicals, spraying foods, dyes or other additives, or fungus, bacteria, or parasites in the intestine that secrete toxins.

Chronic stress which may be mental, emotional, or physical.

Medications such as NSAIDs (ibuprofen type), birth control pills, cortisone, and antibiotics affect digestive health. Also lack of fiber and nutrients like zinc, vitamin C and B vitamins can affect your gut.

Microbial imbalance such as an overgrowth of parasites, bacteria, viruses and fungi which may strain intestinal mucosa.

CROSS REACTIVITY

An **allergen** is a substance that triggers an **allergic reaction** (or a heightened response by the immune system to a relatively harmless invader). Common allergens include milk protein, gluten (wheat, and in many cases also other grains), soy, peanuts, etc. In an allergic reaction the immune system responds quickly, and signs of an allergic reaction can occur within minutes of exposure to an allergen.

Signs of an allergic reaction include: shortness of breath, severe itching, and sudden onset of a rash or hives. Environmental allergens may trigger itchy eyes and runny nose. It is important to understand that food allergy and food intolerance are not the same thing. Food allergies occur when the mast cells begin mistakenly producing excessive histamines and other chemicals in response to harmless allergens.

Food intolerance - is different than an allergy as the reaction is much slower and less intense. It also means that many people are living with food intolerances and may not know it. Symptoms of food intolerance may include inflamed bowel, migraine, skin or joint problems, sleep disorders, weight problems, chronic fatigue and breathing problems.

For the 20% of PPP sufferers with celiac disease or gluten-intolerance/sensitivity (whether diagnosed or not), it is critical to understand the concept of gluten cross-reactivity. Many people following a strict gluten-free diet still suffer from symptoms related to gluten. One reason may be that although the individual is not consuming gluten, their body reacts to specific foods as though they did.

This is called **cross-reactivity**. There are a number of naturally gluten-free foods such as cheese, chocolate and coffee that contain proteins so similar to gluten that your body confuses them for gluten. When you eat these foods your body and immune system react as if you just ate a bowl of whole-wheat pasta. It's estimated that at least half of those who are gluten intolerant are also sensitive to dairy (cheese, yogurt, milk and butter) due to its cross-reactivity with gluten.

It is important to remember it is the immune system rather than the specific food that is the problem. Therefore it is important to heal the digestive tract through nourishing good bacteria, and reducing bad.. When the mucus lining in the gut is healed, you will no longer have a problem with food intolerances as it will no longer leak undigested proteins in to the blood, irritating the immune system.

Below is a list of common foods that cross-react with gluten:

- Amaranth

- Buckwheat

- Chocolate

- Coffee

- Corn

- Dairy i.e. Milk and Cheese (Alpha-Casein, Beta-Casein, Casomorphin, Butyrophilin, Whey Protein)

- Egg

- Hemp

- Millet

- Oats

- Polish wheat

- Potato

- Rice

- Sesame

- Sorghum

- Soy

- Tapioca

- Teff

- Yeast

- Sweeteners, thickeners and other additives (can affect the intestinal flora and cause dysbiosis)

While not all people with gluten sensitivities will be sensitive to the listed foods above, they should definitely be considered as high risk for stimulating the immune system. Just as small amounts of gluten can cause a reaction for people with celiac disease and those sensitive to gluten, a small amount of these foods can trigger inflammation and immune response.

If you suspect you are gluten-intolerant and you are still having health issues even after removing gluten from your diet, try eliminating the above foods for at least two months and see if your symptoms improve.

Make sure you have healed your gut as well. After two months try to reintroduce the restricted food items one at a time to determine which ones you are cross-reacting to, if any at all. If you determine that there are foods that are cross-reactive for you, the treatment is to permanently remove these foods from your diet along with gluten. Remember, that although the cross-reactive foods do not actually contain gluten, your body thinks they do and therefore the inflammation and damage to your body is equal to that of gluten

STRESS / how stress affects our digestion and general health

Stress – everybody talks about it, and most people experience it. It's time for some clear definitions. **Stress** is both a physical and psychological response to a potentially threatening experience. A **stressor** is threat that causes stress, or triggers a stress response. Stressors can include immediate danger, or challenging situations such as an exam, a divorce, or the death of a loved one. There has been little investigation into the role of stress in PPP, but in one small study (Saez-Rodriguez 2002) anxiety scores were found to be higher in patients with PPP than in control patients. The authors suggested that stress and the worsening of PPP may be related. According to this study most autoimmune diseases are triggered by a major stressor. In fact, 80% of people report uncommon emotional stress before disease onset.

A **stress response** (or **fight or flight reaction**), is how our ancestors survived when faced with danger. A cascade of physical changes enable your body to escape danger. Imagine a caveman confronting a saber-toothed tiger – they either run, or they fight. Surging hormones and a boost in available energy make this possible. Modern people still have this same stress response, although our threats have changed. And the way we manage our stress is actually making us sick.

Stress is an unfortunate part of our modern lives, and is an underlying cause of many ailments. I feel it's important to mention the damage stress that causes to our bodies, because many PPP sufferers seem to get flare ups during stressful periods.

The biology of stress

When faced with a stressor, our bodies prepare for either 'fight' or to confront a challenge, or 'flight' and escape a frightening situation. In both cases your body gets ready for a burst of activity – your breathing and heart rate increase, digestion slows and you lose your appetite, and your liver releases glucose to give your body the energy it needs. Emotional reactions can include increased anxiety or aggression as your body prepares to flee or fight.

In a stress response the sympathetic part of the autonomic nervous system becomes activated. Thyroid activity increases, and you may you feel refreshed, alert, warm and creative, and ready to take on a challenge.

Adrenaline and cortisol

During a stress response the body releases **cortisol and adrenaline**. Both hormones help contribute to the body's ability to defend itself, and reduce the sensation of pain, and suppress the immune system (thereby increasing risk of inflammation and infections). The immune system is suppressed as the body channels all available resources to help confront the immediate threat.

Adrenaline gets your body ready to fight or flee, supplying a burst of energy. It quickly increases at the time of danger, and decreases rapidly when the danger is over. **Cortisol** levels can be increased for a long time and make you feel alert, goal orientated, focused, strong and brave (if the adrenal glands are healthy).

Modern stress

Although the physical response to stress has remained the same as our ancestors, the actual stressors have become increasingly complex.

In the past when we lived close to nature, stress was more likely a more single, intense event such as being chased by a predator, fighting, or tribal war. Stressors (such as fleeing a wild animal) were resolved quickly, and adrenaline and cortisol levels rose swiftly to deal with a threat, and then quickly returned to resting levels.

But today stress tends to occur differently. Instead of being chased by an animal, stress is more often triggered by performance requirements at work, relationship problems, financial pressure, or time constraints.

Unfortunately the body cannot distinguish between different stressors. Your basic stress response still works the same way as when our Stone Age forefathers were preparing for flight or fight. The problem with modern stress is the stressors do not resolve quickly. Problems at work, in relationships, or financial strain linger in your life, creating a more or less permanent state of heightened stress response.

Even the physical activity that the body uses in order to face a stressful situation is missing if you're not exercising enough. This contributes to stress hormones remaining in the body even longer.

Long term stress

Only now are we beginning to recognize the negative health effects of long term stress. If faced with constant or recurring stressors (such as workplace conflicts) the body's stress response remains active and has no opportunity to return to normal levels. You're in a near permanent 'fight or flight' response.

Over time, repeated activation of the stress response takes a toll on the body. Research suggests that prolonged stress contributes to high blood pressure, promotes the formation of artery-clogging deposits, and causes brain changes that may contribute to anxiety, depression, and addiction. Other research suggests that chronic stress may also contribute to obesity, both directly (causing people to eat more) or indirectly (decreasing sleep and exercise).

Recall that anxiety and aggression are part of the basic stress response. Another response is a completely focusing on a single task, or tunnel vision. You lose sight of the bigger picture and have a diminished ability to view things from a broader perspective. In this case, the little things become a big deal. Increased anxiety, aggression (or irritability) and this diminished perspective can create or perpetuate even more conflicts, thereby exacerbating the prolonged stress response. So if relationship conflicts are stressing you out, the stress response itself will cause you to be anxious or irritable, and to focus on 'the little things', which in turn leads to even more fighting.

It's a modern dilemma. You have to work hard just to keep up. For many this means they rarely feel at ease when not occupied or doing something they think is of importance. I used to be like that. I always made sure I filled my diary and kept busy. For most people night time is the only time we actually set aside to rest and to recover, and we might not even manage to do that.

The importance of rest

The parasympathetic part of the autonomic nervous system is activated only during time of rest, such as when you meditate, chill out, do something enjoyable, think positive and loving thoughts, and when you digest food. This may also explain why many become tired after a meal. You digest food for many hours each day; this requires that you give yourself room to rest.

Television viewing and Facebook are not part of resting as they create a measurable stress response in the brain. Additionally, you remain preoccupied with processing external messages (often frightening and negative ones) which prevents you from going within and finding inner peace.

The importance of sleep

Sleep plays a vital role in good health and well-being, but everyone's individual sleep needs vary. In general, most healthy adults are built for 16 hours of wakefulness and need an average of eight hours of sleep a night. However, some individuals are able to function without sleepiness or drowsiness after as little as six hours of sleep.

As Chris Kresser stated in his blog, "Sleep is absolutely essential for basic maintenance and repair of the neurological, endocrine, immune, musculoskeletal and digestive systems. The hormone melatonin naturally increases after sundown and during the night in a normal circadian rhythm, which increases immune cytokine function and helps protect us against infection. (This is why you're so likely to get a cold or flu after not sleeping well for a few nights.)"

Thinking back to the time I was sick; I rarely got more than five hours of sleep at night, this was partly due to my daughter waking me up for nightly feeding, and again, me not looking after myself. Lesson learned.

What happens to digestion during times of stress?

When you are exposed to stress for an extended period of time your thyroid and adrenal glands work hard producing high levels of adrenaline and cortisol.

Eventually, they become overworked and slow down. You might feel exhausted and unable to meet the increasingly stressful demands.

If you are not listening to your body's signals when this is happening there's a chance you might compensate for the energy shortage and feelings of stress by consuming alcohol, dairy products, sugar, wheat flour, caffeine, chocolate, nicotine, or salt to provide a sense of relaxation and enjoyment.

The problem with excessive consumption of these substances is that over time they fatigue your entire organ and glandular systems. This exacerbates the problem even more.

The thyroid and the adrenal glands also indirectly control the gastric acid production in the stomach. When these glands are not working efficiently, gastric acid production will decrease. This contributes to a reduced ability to absorb nutrients, especially B vitamins, folic acid, vitamin K2 and iron. In addition it compromises the breakdown of protein-based foods.

As mentioned previously, if gastric acid levels are too low the esophagus may not close completely, creating symptoms of heartburn and acid reflux. This is especially problematic if the low gastric acid levels are misdiagnosed and treated with conventional medication for acid reflux (excessive gastric acid).

As gastric acid is an essential first step in the digestion process, low levels of gastric acid impair your body's ability to break down food in the stomach, and the food enters the intestines less digested than it should be. When the food we eat arrives into the intestine in this condition, the body must take rescue measures.

Changes in available enzymes and the mobility of the intestine (as stress slows the digestive tract) affect your body's ability to digest food.

Recall that in normal digestion your intestinal tract is filled with bacteria that help break food down, and the balance of 'good bacteria' to 'bad' is essential. But if food continues to enter the digestive tract as in an undigested state, it will change the balance of the gut flora.

Not only antibiotics, candida, gluten and biofilms disrupt the gut flora and your body's ability to digest food, but also stress.

Stress is a silent killer in our busy modern times. Elevated hormone levels, hypertension, clogged arteries, obesity, anxiety, addiction, and depression – long term stress is killing us.

Actively trying to destress is essential, and may be achieved through rest, exercise, and social support. Whether chatting with friends, a yoga class, or making sure you get enough sleep – you may find a way that works best for you. For me, walking is an amazing form of relaxation; I love to be outdoors in the fresh air with my own thoughts. Its exercise and meditation rolled into one.

"Healing is a matter of time, but it is sometimes also a matter of opportunity"
— Hippocrates

Part 2

WHAT TRIGGERS PPP? / Getting to the Root of the Situation

Through modern medicine we have been lulled into the belief that pills and medicines are the single cure-all for everything. In reality it is our own immune system that does the actual job of keeping us healthy, medicine just helps it along. If our immune system isn't working properly we have a diminished defense against inflammatory conditions which may occur in the body. **As in most cases of autoimmune disease, there are no pills that can cure the chronic inflammation that causes the disease in the first place**, apart from biologics that might suppress the symptoms for a while.

Doctors are trained to identify diseases based on where symptoms show in your body. If you have asthma it's considered a lung problem, if you have rheumatoid arthritis it must be a joint problems, if you have acne, doctors see it as a skin problems, if you are overweight you must have a metabolic problem and so on.

Modern medicine has a compartmentalized view of the human body, and doctors who look at health this way are both right and wrong. Sometimes the underlying causes of your symptoms do have some relationship to their location, but that's far from the whole picture.

What's your trigger? One or all of them?

To be able to heal your PPP you need to determine what your trigger is. In my case my PPP was caused by a combination of factors. I smoked during my youth, I went through a very stressful time in both in work and at home, I had taken several courses of antibiotics after repeated strep throat infections; resulting in imbalanced gut flora. My diet consisted mostly of bread, pasta, pizza, and a lot of biscuits and sweets; this lead to continuous yeast infections that wouldn't go away when treated. I can only assume I had candida as well.

Smoking

As mentioned in the Swedish case study, smoking is a significant factor in developing PPP. For someone with PPP, the most important thing is to stop smoking; and if you are not able to give up cigarettes completely, at least cut down.

Although PPP will not go away if stopping smoking is the only thing you do, by stop smoking the abnormal cell activity in the parathyroid gland will hopefully go back to normal so it can produce parathyroid hormone. The parathyroid hormone is the hormone which lets your body know it has to pull calcium from your bones in order to start making more activated vitamin D in order to absorb more calcium in the gut.

Gluten

We know nearly 20% of people suffering with PPP are gluten intolerant; this number may be much higher as it very difficult to test people as gluten intolerance may be thought of as a range, rather than an absolute. Some people may tolerant gluten, but are still sensitive to wheat or the gluten protein. The only way to effectively determine the gluten tolerance is to exclude gluten from your diet completely. By doing so you will heal the lining in your gut and give your body a chance to repair.

Because there is no way to be absolutely sure if wheat or gluten is the culprit, my recommendation is to exclude gluten for at least three months. It might seem hard initially, but for me once I got in to it and found alternatives, I felt much better.

Bacterial Overgrowth

If a strep throat infection triggered your PPP, it is very likely your gut flora is impaired due to the antibiotics you were given. It is also probable that you have biofilms that inhibits the gut's ability to absorb vitamins and minerals. The bad bacteria and biofilms also displace the good bacteria and impair their ability to create the vitamins K2 and D3.

Vitamins K2 and D3 are important for properly distributing calcium in your body. This is crucial for PPP sufferers who have increased of calcium levels in the body. Calcium is also a significant promoter of biofilm formation in most pathogenic bacterial species, and also promotes formation of candida albicans biofilms. The way I removed my biofilms was to take 5 milliliters of colloidal silver orally every day, and I still take it.

It is very difficult to break down biofilms, but in a study from 2005 researchers found that colloidal silver can break down biofilms caused by the bacteria staphylococcus epidermis within hours.

Colloidal silver also kills parasites, fungus and the bad bacteria in the gut, making it an effective way to restore imbalanced gut flora, only as long as you supplement with prebiotics. I have read about people having success breaking down biofilms with apple cider vinegar and enzymes such as nattokinase, serrapeptase, and lumbrokinase, but I don't know how effective this is as I have not tried it myself. During my healing process I also supplemented with **vitamin K2, D3, biotin, good prebiotics, zinc, colostrum and chlorella**.

Vitamin and Mineral Deficient

During my time of healing I was determined to boost my immune system and return to my pre-PPP health. I felt that if I was able to wreck my immune system by poor life style choices, there must be a way to restore it by changing my bad habits. Everything inside our bodies is made up of cells, and for the body to function properly, every single cell must perform their individual jobs to the best of their ability. Our cells need essential nutrients to thrive and function optimally.

Throughout my PPP journey I researched nutrition and completed a course on the subject. I changed my diet by cutting out all sugars, aside from the natural sugars found in fruit and vegetables. I also stopped eating gluten.

I can't say I followed a specific diet, but I'd say it's a mix of the GAPS, FODMAP, LCHF (Low Carb, High Fat), Paleo, and the anti-candida diet. I also started to juice green juices and drank a big glass of wonderful vitamin and mineral-filled cocktails every morning. Drinking green juices are a great way for your body to get all the vitamins and minerals quickly in to the system.

Diets can be very individualized; whatever works for me doesn't necessarily work for somebody else. We are all different and my advice is for to use trial and error to determine which foods are potentially triggering inflammation and sensitivities, and eliminate them accordingly.

But the general rule is: No sugar, No Gluten, No processed foods, No additives, preservatives, artificial colours, or flavours. And you should eat only real whole foods that are preferably organic, and consume alcohol in moderation.

Stress

As mentioned before, autoimmunity occurs when the immune system becomes confused. Your body is fighting something, anything from an infection, a toxin (poison), an allergen, or perhaps a constant supply of the hormone cortisol caused by stress.

I knew I needed to do something about my stress levels. I woke up every morning with a racing pulse, shortness of breath, and a pain in my heart. As a blessing in disguise I was laid off at work due to the employer's relocation. I was given a six months' notice, which gave me plenty of time to find a new job. The new job was far more relaxed and better paid; for the first time in a long time I could breathe normally again, my stress levels definitely decreased.

Interesting enough, although I have been PPP-free for the past three years, a few months ago when I went through a stressful period four new blisters formed on the palm of my hand. I could hardly see them, but I freaked out. I phoned in sick and stayed home for a couple days to unwind. I kept taking baths with loads of Epsom salt (Epsom salts contain magnesium sulphate) during my time off, and interestingly enough the blisters never developed in to a PPP outbreak. Thankfully they just faded away.

SIX STEPS TO TREAT PPP

1. Do some investigative work to determine if you have a hidden infection like fungus (candida overgrowth), viruses, bacteria, or parasites that can cause biofilms. Your best bet is to try to improve your gut health through removing contributing factors, trying to break down biofilms and restore good bacteria.

2. Do even more investigative work to determine whether you have hidden food allergies by trial and error testing of sensitivity to particular foods, especially gluten. The only way to assess gluten sensitivity is through an elimination diet.

3. Heal your gut. Stop eating gluten!

Remember the general rule: No sugar, No Gluten, No processed foods, No additives, preservatives, artificial colors, or flavors. And only eat real whole foods that are preferably organic, and consume alcohol in moderation.

4. Supplement with nutrients such as zinc, magnesium, Vitamin K2 together with D3, biotin, colostrum and probiotics to naturally boost and calm down the immune system.

5. Exercise regularly, as it has natural anti-inflammatory actions within the body. A 30 minute walk every day is a great way to boost your immune system and minimize the effects of chronic stress.

6. Deal with stress, and make sure stress management is part of your daily health regime. Say no, prioritize, and do stress-busting activities such as yoga, massage, exercise, and Epsom salt baths (that are full of magnesium) to counteract the long term stress response that triggers the release of the hormone cortisol.

Putting all the pieces together

To target a complex autoimmune illness like PPP, and begin to restore your health and repair imbalanced gut flora, you will need to make changes on multiple levels. The tricky part is to know what your triggers are, as they are hard to test and diagnose.

The first step is to take care of nutrition and avoid any food that can potentially cause problems such as an allergic response, sensitivities, or a leaking gut. This includes any grains, sugar, processed food, and for some people, nightshade vegetables, dairy, nuts and seeds.

Eat a well-balanced diet full of all the nutrients the body needs to function. I highly recommend having a green juice every day. Some of the essential nutrients are zinc, vitamin D3, vitamin K2, magnesium, vitamin C, and biotin. Those vitamins also happen to be low in most people's diets, so make sure you include these supplements.

The next step is to try to disrupt bacterial biofilms present in the gut with multiple strategies. These include avoiding calcium and iron, as these minerals are used by bacteria to form biofilms. For some, taking special enzymes on an empty stomach has been proved successful. I recommend natural anti-fungal, antiviral and antibacterial agents such as colloidal silver; other natural antibiotics and antibacterial agents include olive leaf extract, citrus seed extracts, kolorex, iodine, bee propolis, Manuka honey, oregano oil, undecenoic acid and caprylic acid.

As the third step, it's absolutely essential to rebuild healthy gut flora with a high dose of beneficial bacteria. The right type of bacteria to take will depend on your specific problems, but usually **lactobacillus bacteria** is a very good starting point. You can also buy or make your own fermented vegetables such as sauerkraut, which are full of natural probiotics.

Finally, you need to actively manage the stress in your life. Chronic stress will undermine all your efforts for improving your health. You need to include exercise and stress management as part of your daily regime. Say no to what you can while your body is healing; this is the time to focus on your needs. You only have one life to live, and it's yours to make the best of it. Nothing else matters.

During my healing process I followed all the steps listed above, and it took about two and a half months for my skin to heal and my PPP to be completely cleared, so be patient and stick with it. I also want to mention that during these months I still would get PPP outbreaks, but every time they happened on a smaller scale, until eventually it all stopped.

HOW TO IMPROVE YOUR IMMUNE SYSTEM THROUGH DIET

As you know, everything inside our bodies and the skin that surrounds us is made of cells. So for the body to function properly, the cells need to function too. It is crucial to give the cells and the good bacteria in the gut the nutrients they need to function optimally.

The only way to do this is to eat a nutritious diet and remove the foods that are not beneficial, as they say, **'you are what you eat'** – and poor quality nutrition affects the very basic structure and functioning of your body. A diet high in convenience foods may taste appealing, but there is little for cells to develop and grow from, and very few available nutrients for your body to use as fuel.

At first, it might seem overwhelming to cut things you love out, and it will be challenging to figure out appropriate substitutions. My advice is to start with baby steps, and not do everything at once. Look at it as a long term lifestyle change, where the goal is to become well and heal from PPP.

Start with cutting out processed foods for a couple of weeks to get in to the habit of cooking yourself, and move on to remove all sugars from your diet (including sugary drinks), finally cut out gluten as well. These changes will be challenging, especially at first as you break bad habits and replace them with new ones. But I promise you, once your body begins to feel better, you will want to continue.

I recommend juicing daily (green fresh juices, not processed fruit juices) as soon as possible. (If you don't have a juicer, seriously consider buying one as it can become quite expensive to buy green juice every day.) When you start changing your diet, be sure to begin a daily mineral and vitamin supplement regime. I recommend colloidal silver, zinc, vitamin D3, vitamin K2, biotin, magnesium, chlorella, colostrum and probiotics.

ALPHABET SOUP: AN OVERVIEW OF SPECIFIC DIETS – GAPS, PALEO, HCFC, FODMAP AND MORE

Diets high in fat and low in carbs and Paleolithic diets has never been as popular as they are now. There are thousands of anecdotal stories from people who successfully managed to heal themselves from disease and to lose weight by following these type of diets (including me!). There are also many cookbooks available supporting these healing diets such as GAPS (Gut and Psychology Syndrome), PALEO, The Candida Diet, LCHF (Low Carb High Fat), FODMAP (The IBS diet).

These diets are all very similar as they all involve eating real food and remove the foods causing inflammation and damage to the body, as well as cutting out foods that have no nutritional value. If you suspect leaky gut, unbalanced gut flora, candida or an allergy to a particular food, you might find it's overwhelming figuring out what to eat and what not to; following an established diet can be very helpful. In the table below I've summarized the most popular healing diets to-date.

GAPS Summary

The GAPS diet is a comprehensive healing protocol developed by Dr. Natasha Campbell-McBride, a neurologist and nutritionist who specializes in healing of issues like autism spectrum disorders, ADD/ADHD, dyspraxia, dyslexia and schizophrenia by treating the root cause of many of these disorders.

Candida Diet Summary

Because the Candida fungus loves sugar, a completely sugar-free diet (including removing fruit) is the best way to go to get rid of yeast over growth. Switching to a low-sugar diet deprives the Candida of the food that it needs to grow and spread through your digestive system.

FODMAP Diet Summary

The FODMAP diet was developed by Peter Gibson and Susan Shepherd as a treatment for IBS in 1999, and has since become very popular. They mapped all the common foods we eat.

FODMAPs is an acronym referring to Fermentable Oligosaccharides, Disaccharides, Monosaccharides and Polyols. These are complex names for a collection of molecules found in food that can be poorly absorbed by some people. Any FODMAPs that are not absorbed in the small intestine pass into the large intestine, where bacteria ferment them. The resultant production of gas contributes to bloating and flatulence. Most individuals do not suffer significant symptoms, but some may suffer IBS-type symptoms. For individuals with IBS-type symptoms, restriction of FODMAP intake has been found to result in great improvements.

LCHF Diet Summary

Low-carbohydrate (low carb) diets are dietary programs that restrict carbohydrate consumption, often for the treatment of obesity or diabetes. Foods high in easily digestible carbohydrates (such as sugars, bread, and pasta) are limited or replaced by lower carb foods, such as proteins or vegetables. Ideal substitutions are foods containing a higher percentage of fats and moderate protein (such as meats, poultry, fish, shellfish, eggs, cheese, nuts, and seeds) and other foods low in carbohydrates (such as most salad vegetables such as spinach, kale, chard and collards); although other vegetables and fruits (especially berries) are often allowed.

PALEO Diet Summary

The Paleolithic diet, also known as the paleo diet or caveman diet, is a diet based on the foods our ancient ancestors likely ate, such as meat, nuts and berries. This diet excludes foods they didn't have access to, like dairy.

The diet is based on several premises. Proponents of the diet state that during the Paleolithic era — a period lasting around 2.5 million years that ended about 10,000 years ago, with the advent of agriculture and domestication of animals — humans evolved nutritional needs specific to the foods available at that time, and that the nutritional needs of modern humans remain best adapted to the diet of their Paleolithic ancestors.

Colour Codes	Ok To Eat	Not Ok	Can Eat in small amounts			
Diet	Anti Histamin	GAPS	FODMAP	LCHF	Paleo	Anticandida
Drinks						
Organic Coffee						
Organic Coconut Milk						
Water with lemon						
Unsweetend Milk from nuts						
Soya Milk						
Milk free from lactos						
Rice Milk						
Sweetend drinks/Sodas						
Energy Drinks						
Fruit Juices						
Red Wine						
Liquer (vodka, Gin, Whiskey, Single Malt)						
Foodstuff	Anti Histamin	GAPS	FODMAP	LCHF	Paleo	Anticandida
Vegetables						
Alfalfa sprouts, Ainer						
Sellerie, Fennel						
Asparagus, Avocado, Cucumber						
Spinach, Kale						
Broccoli, Cauliflower						
Carrots, Leek, Parsley, Green Beans, Artichokes, Squash						
Onion, Aubergine, Peppers, Peas, Scallion						
Raw Kale, Raw Spinach, Pumpkins, Beats						
Sweetcorn						
Vegetable Oil and Fats	Anti Histamin	GAPS	FODMAP	LCHF	Paleo	Anticandida
MCT Oil, Egg Yolks, Coconut Oil, Avocado Oil, Cocoa Butter						
Organic Butter, Fish Oil, Krill Oil						
Bacon Fat, Palm Oil, Olive Oil						
Duck Fat, Lard						
Butter from Non Grass Fed Cows						

Peanut Butter, Rapseed, Sunflower and other Vegtable Oils						
Margarine, Artificial Trans Fats, Oils from GMO Crops						
Nuts and Legumes	Anti Histamin	GAPS	FODMAP	LCHF	Paleo	Anticandida
Coconuts, Olives						
Kidney Beans						
Almonds, Cashew Nuts, Hazelnut, Pecan Nuts, Macadamia Nuts						
Chestnut, Walnuts						
Hummus, Dried Peas						
Pulse, Dried Beans and Lentils, Peanuts						
Pistachio, Pine Nuts, Sprouted Legumes						
Soya Beans						
Dairy	Anti Histamin	GAPS	FODMAP	LCHF	Paleo	Anticandida
Organic Ghee, Organic Butter						
Homemade Yogurt						
Soft Cheese						
Creame Fraiche						
Cream 40% Fat						
Milk (Alll kinds)						
Sour Cream						
Cheese						
Brie Cheese, Camembert etc…						
Quark						
Protein	Anti Histamin	GAPS	FODMAP	LCHF	Paleo	Anticandida
Beef, Pork, Chicken, Fish from good sources						
Organic Eggs						
Whey and Casein Protein						
Hemp Protein						
Pea Protein						
Rice Protein						
Soy Protein						
Egg Protein						
Starches	Anti Histamin	GAPS	FODMAP	LCHF	Paleo	Anticandida
Sweet Potatos, Carrots, Pumpkins						
White Rice, Cassava						
Brown Rice						
Banana						

Black Rice						
Potatos						
Bulgur, Buckwheat						
Oat, Quinia						
Wheat and other grains, Gluten Free Products						

Fruit and Berries	Anti Histamin	GAPS	FODMAP	LCHF	Paleo	Anticandida
Blueberries, Raspberries, Lemon, Lime, Strawberries, Avocado, Coconuts						
Pineapple, Grape Fruit						
Apples, Aprocots, Cherries, Kiwi, Figs, Pears, Plums, Nectarine						
Passion Fruit, Grapes, Mango, Melons, Papaya, Dates						
Dried Fruit						
Canned Fruits, Jam, Marmelade						

Spice and Flavouring	Anti Histamin	GAPS	FODMAP	LCHF	Paleo	Anticandida
Applecider Vinegar						
Seasalt, Himalaya Salt						
Ginger						
Oregano, Tumeric, Lavendel						
Cinnamon						
Garlic, Black Pepper, Paprika						
Tofu, Miso						
Premixed Dressings and spices, MSG, Hydrolysed Gluten E620 and other E-Numbers						

Sweeteners	Anti Histamin	GAPS	FODMAP	LCHF	Paleo	Anticandida
Xylitol, Stevia, Erythritol						
Sorbitol, Maltitol and other Sugar Alcohol						
Raw Honey						
Coconut Sugar						
Fructos, Fruit Juice from Concentrate, fructose syrup						
Aspartame, Sucralose, Acesulfame K						
White Sugar, Brown Sugar, Regular Honey, Agave						

SUPPLEMENTS – THE HOWS AND WHYS

Apart from removing sugar, gluten and processed foods from your diet, eating only real foods, it is equally important to supplement with certain vitamins to help the body kick start the healing process. I'm a firm believer that if you eat the right types of food, you normally don't have to supplement with vitamins, especially if you are juicing greens. There are some supplements though, that should be part of your daily healing regime; the reason being that some of them are not available through food, and for others, most people with an unbalanced gut flora lack.

Why Colloidal Silver?

Colloidal silver may be controversial for some people as there are no in vivo studies (studies made on humans inside the body) but only in vitro studies (studies in test tubes) to prove it actually works. Colloidal silver supplements harness the antibacterial properties of silver, while reducing health risks. There are millions of people worldwide using colloidal silver supplements daily (including myself) who can report on the enormous health benefits it has. In our family we use it for budding ear infections, colds, warts, cuts, sore throats, as well as taking it orally – we find it works like magic.

Silver has long been recognized in recorded history as having germicidal properties. In 69 B.C. silver nitrate was described in the ancient pharmaceutical texts. In ancient Greece, Rome, Phoenicia, and Macedonia, silver was used extensively to manage many immune challenges. From the time man first learned to work with silver, he has known that it delayed the spoilage of foods and that it reduced the symptoms of illness. Hippocrates, the "Father of Medicine," used silver and stated that it promoted tissue repair, at that time it was a notable topical aid. In the days before refrigeration, people tossed a silver coin in a bucket of milk to keep it from spoiling.

The use of silver as an antibiotic gave way to the convenience of sulfa drugs and then eventually to the use of penicillin. Originally the drugs were highly effective and easy to use; now we face antibiotic-resistant bacteria from overuse. It is important to note that bacteria do not generally develop resistance to silver unless the bacteria have a very thick wall that does not absorb it. Colloidal silver is effective against most gram positive and gram negative bacteria.

Silver ions bind to cell walls and are then absorbed into the single-cell bacteria or fungus where they interfere with the cellular energy production and kill the organism. The fermentation system of energy production used by these single cell organisms is different than the aerobic energy producing system of human cells, which are not so affected by silver. This shows that silver is not toxic to human cells and a great way to get rid of the bad bacteria, yeast in your gut.

There are warnings about colloidal silver all over the Internet causing an irreversible condition called **argyria** (your skin turns blue when you ingest large quantities of silver salts or silver particles). It is important to understand that argyria is caused by misuse of cheaper products marketed as colloidal silver mixed with salts and protein, and not real colloidal silver. Colloidal silver produced with high voltage technology does not cause argyria. .

A good colloidal silver product will also have third-party product research backing up any claims. Make sure the colloidal silver that you use does not contain any additional ingredients such as salts or proteins. These ingredients provide an unstable solution. Because there are so many different types of colloidal silver on the market, I advise you do your own research about any colloidal silver product you are considering taking.

Because colloidal silver is such a potent antibacterial agent, it is advisable to supplement with probiotics during use, even though there is no current proof that a properly made colloidal silver will harm gut flora. Unlike antibiotics that wipe out both the bad and the good gut bacteria, silver maintains a balance of intestinal microorganisms. Because silver is quickly absorbed in the upper GI tract, little gets through to cause problems for the beneficial bacteria in the small intestine and colon. But the bottom line is you will need to do your own research with regards to colloidal silver use, to determine if is right for you.

Reported benefits of colloidal silver include:

• Colloidal silver improves and maintains a healthy immune system, and helps optimize gut flora balance through breaking down biofilms.

• It is a powerful antibiotic, with antibacterial, anti-parasitic, and antimicrobial qualities, and has been uses as purifier and a topical antiseptic and antifungal agent for centuries.

• Colloidal silver is easily digestible and quickly absorbed, with no known contradictions to medications

• It has been used to relieve eye irritation and treat sun spots, candida, dental infections, MRSA infections and urinary tract infections. Colloidal silver fights the common cold and virtually all strains of the flu.

D3 and Vitamin K2

Most people do not have a shortage of calcium in the body, and for those of us with PPP, we have too much calcium. The big problem that due to the absence of other nutrients (especially of vitamin K2 and D3), excess calcium ends up in the wrong places in the body.

This leads to the 'calcium paradox', where there is a deficiency of calcium in the bones, while at the same time there's a surplus of calcium in other tissues, including blood vessels. When calcium is stored in the blood vessel walls, they become narrower and more rigid. The missing factor is vitamin K2.

Why Vitamin K2?

Most people are unaware of the health benefits of vitamin K2. The K vitamins have been underrated and misunderstood until very recently in both the scientific community and the general public. It was commonly believed that the benefits of vitamin K are limited to its role in blood clotting, and that vitamins K1 and K2 are simply different forms of the same vitamin.

Vitamin K2 is a very important micronutrient and most people are deficient, especially those with a disrupted gut flora, because vitamin K2 is normally produced by gut flora. Vitamin K2 also prevents against vitamin D toxicity and activates the proteins created by vitamin D and vitamin A for proper utilization of calcium.

Some food sources include butter from grass-fed and pastured animals, goose liver, duck liver and egg yolks. Some fermented products like natto and cheeses such as Edam cheese are also high in the MK-7 form of vitamin K2.

Why Vitamin D3?

Vitamin D produced in the skin when we are exposed to the sun. The problem here in the northern hemisphere is the sun is only strong enough in the middle of the day and during the summer months, and applying a high SPF sun protection doesn't help. Unfortunately we get very little vitamin D from food. The result is that many people living in the North (perhaps most) are deficient in vitamin D.

Vitamin D is unique among all the vitamins. It is a steroid hormone just like our sex hormones and affects hundreds of genes in most cells of the body. Potentially, a deficiency in this vitamin can affect the health in countless ways.

Current research suggests that vitamin D deficiency plays a role in a variety of inflammation diseases such as seasonal depressions, cancer, heart disease, osteoporosis, autism, general pain, fibromyalgia, and obesity. Current recommendations are to take 1000 iu (international units) of vitamin D3 daily.

Why Colostrum (Lactoferrin)?

Colostrum is the first milk secreted by the mother before the regular breast milk develops . This is something that all newborn mammals naturally produce. There's an abundance of colostrum in the first milk the cow produces after calving. It contains over 90 known components and is full of bacterial binding immunoglobulins, antibiotic acting proteins and growth factors. It also contains the perfect balance of vitamins, minerals and amino acids. Colostrum from cows and humans are similar in composition, but research shows that the cow has four times more powerful immune enhancing factors than colostrum from humans.

The immune enhancing factors in Colostrum (Lactoferrin) can help to:

• Balance and support a healthy immune system

• Balance an overactive immune system associated with autoimmune diseases

• Support an underactive immune system

• Regulate the thymus gland due its polypeptides rich in proline.

• Combat harmful invaders such as viruses, bacteria, yeast and fungi. Colostrum contains over 20 antibodies to specific pathogens such as E. coli, salmonella, rotavirus, candida, streptococcus, staphylococcus, H pylori and cryptosporidium.

The growth factors in colostrum provide essential building blocks in the newborn for the growth of the cells, muscles, tissue, bone, and cartilage. During aging the body produce fewer of these growth factors.

These growth factors in Colostrum (Lactoferrin) contribute to the following:

• Increasing the level of thin tissue

- Supporting wound healing

- Helping regulate neurotransmitters that control the mood and emotional state

- Helping the body to burn fat instead of muscle tissue while fasting

- Assisting in the regulation of blood glucose levels and chemicals necessary for proper brain function

- Repairing our RNA and DNA

Toxins like alcohol, smoking and carcinogens all weaken the immune response; colostrum helps the body restore a normal immune response in both young children and adults. Colostrum acts as a prebiotic, contributing to healthy gut flora and boosting the immune system, as it is also rich in bacterial binding immunoglobulin, antibiotic-acting proteins as well as growth factors. It also assists in the binding of pathogens to the intestinal wall so that they cannot spread. Colostrum has a strong anti-bacterial properties, destroying opportunistic bacteria and biofilms.

Studies indicate that colostrum can be effective in treating conditions such as indigestion, inflammatory bowel disease, ulcers, and damage from NSAIDs (anti-inflammatory drugs), as well as chemotherapy induced inflammation in the intestinal mucosa.

Why Magnesium?

Magnesium is a mineral that is important for more than 300 enzymes to work properly, and is essential for proper digestion and elimination. A magnesium deficiency contributes to delays in bowel emptying; this results in malabsorption and constipation, and subsequent gut flora problems.

Magnesium is also important for proper and restorative sleep, vitamin D function and immune system function. Magnesium is essential in preventing allergies, detoxifying, improving skin quality and promoting relaxation. I don't supplement with magnesium, but do take baths with Epsom salt (pure magnesium) and soak for 30 minutes once a week. Avocados and green juice are an excellent source of magnesium.

Why the mineral Zinc?

Zinc deficiency is a contributing factor in the development of psoriasis. There are studies that have found lower levels of zinc in people with psoriasis compared to people without. Zinc deficiency often occurs in people who are gluten sensitive or have dairy intolerance, and the lack of this mineral is a marker that something is wrong. One sign of zinc deficiency is white spots, stripes, pits or brittleness in the nails.

Although most doctors will not immediately suggest a check of zinc levels, deficiency indicates greater problems, and often occurs when the intestinal mucosa has been damaged, such as by gluten. Importantly, the body requires more zinc when ill or exposed to stress.

Symptoms of zinc deficiency include:

• Skin conditions like psoriasis, eczema, blemishes, acne, slow healing of wounds, ruptures in the skin, dandruff, hair loss, white spots on the nails and sores on the shins.

• Impaired cognitive functioning and altered mental states as apathy, irritability, depression, aggression and poor learning ability.

• Widespread health problems, including visual disturbances, circulatory and blood diseases, cancer, and certain kidney and liver problems, and indigestion due to reduced production of digestive enzymes, and an increase in gastric ulcers.

Also, hormonal problems such as diabetes, impaired fertility and menstrual difficulties, reduced milk production in nursing women, fetal birth defects, and disturbances in development and growth.

• Impaired taste and smell ability, bad breath, bad taste in mouth, foul body odor, a white coating on the tongue, weight loss, fatigue, and increased susceptibility to infections. A strong desire for salt and carbohydrates are very common in zinc deficiency.

Why Biotin?

Intestinal bacteria normally produce enough biotin for the body, but with impaired gut flora this is not happening. **There are many anecdotal stories of people who managed to put their PPP in remission by taking biotin supplements.**

Signs of biotin deficiency include depression, panic attacks, hallucinations, muscle pain, dry skin, anemia, heart problems, nausea, severe fatigue, poor appetite, rash, hair loss and hypersensitivity to touch.

• Biotin support B cell and immune system function and helps maintain healthy skin, hair, and nails, as well as sweat glands, nerves, bone marrow and endocrine health.

• Biotin required for normal digestion of proteins, fats and B vitamins. It is also necessary for gluconeogenesis (conversion of amino acids to glucose in the liver), and insulin production and release. Biotin and acts as a coenzyme in several metabolic reactions.

• Biotin is produced by the body in a well-functioning digestive system with good intestinal flora, and helps support intestinal health. Biotin will counter the opportunistic candida fungus, supplementing with biotin may give relief to candida symptoms.

Those with an increased risk of developing biotin deficiency are people who are taking antibiotics, smokers, the elderly, athletes and epileptics. A caution for people who eat more than a raw egg a day, or consume large quantities of alcohol – both alcohol and egg whites contain avidin, this prevents the absorption of biotin.

Why Enzymes?

Enzymes are small proteins and perform vital functions in digestion, metabolism and immune function.

Enzymes have several proven therapeutic effects:

• They breaks down complex proteins like viruses and bacteria.

• They can reduce swelling and inflammation, and accelerate healing.

• They assist in reducing body weight through fat-degradation.

In addition to your body's own enzyme production, we use enzymes naturally found in raw foods. However these are destroyed when food is heated. Therefore, most foods contain very few vital enzymes. A deficiency in essential enzymes impairs digestion and nutrient absorption. It also increases toxic load in the body and reduces the protection against infections.

Food rich in enzymes include:

• Fresh pineapple

- Wheat grass juice

- Sauerkraut

- Pickled vegetables

- Freshly ground raw beef

Why Probiotics?

Probiotics are defined by WHO as 'live microorganisms which, when ingested in sufficient amount, have beneficial effects on the host'. Lactic acid bacteria isolated from the human gastrointestinal system, plant material or foods are usually used as probiotics.

Probiotics were discovered by a Russian scientist who noticed that some groups of people living in the Bulgarian countryside and Russian steppes lived longer than others. He found a connection with their consumption of milk fermented with lactic acid bacteria. Now probiotics are often used in fermented dairy products or food supplements.

Probiotic organisms are intended to support the bacterial flora already in your digestive tract.

Commonly used supplements include organisms from the lactobacillus, bifidobacterium, enterococcus, and streptococcus species. All of them produce lactic acid.

An essential part of digestive health, and promoting a healthy immune system, probiotics actively defend against harmful bacteria by creating barriers, attaching directly to hostile cells, or by changing the pH of their environment.

Probiotics support the body's production of vitamins B1, B3, B6, B12, and vitamin K. Probiotics also produce various enzymes, and facilitate carbohydrate breakdown and energy release. Probiotics strengthen the immune system by activating immune cells, and increasing the production of immune factors. It has also been found that probiotics can reduce the inflammation and hypersensitivity response in allergic reactions.

Why Chlorella?

Chlorella is a type of algae – a green, single cell freshwater microalgae that's loaded with nutrients. It contains more nucleic acids than any other food, which gives it a lot of energy producing potential. It is a great supplement to boost any diet lacking in green vegetables. It has a wide variety of useful nutritional applications, which include supporting natural detoxification, digestive health, immune function, inflammation reduction, antioxidant function, estrogen balance, cholesterol metabolism, and circulation.

Studies have found chlorella can reduce inflammation, boost immune system functioning, and improve your body's response to stress.

Chlorella contains more chlorophyll than most plants, along with an impressive array of vitamins and minerals

(A, D, E, K1, beta carotene, lutein, B vitamins, iron, calcium, potassium, phosphorus, magnesium, and zinc) which are crucial for cells to function properly.

Why Green Juices?

Green juices are made with mostly vegetables and some fruits, often containing as much as a day's worth of veggies in a single serving. Filled with antioxidants, phytochemicals, minerals and vitamins, green juices are ideal for providing the nutrition your body needs.

When vegetables are juiced, the natural sugars in the vegetable are separated from the pulp, which is where the fiber is located. You may feel a "pump" of energy once those natural sugars get into your bloodstream and your glucose levels are raised. Green juices usually start with fresh vegetables such as spinach, kale, broccoli or others as your base.

In a study published in the journal "Cell" in 2011, researchers at the Babraham Institute in Cambridge, England, reported that cruciferous vegetables such as bok choy and broccoli contain a compound that boosts immunity and provides an extra layer of protection to cells in the body.

I tend to drink my green juice on an empty stomach in the morning—because the nutrients are going straight to my digestive tract. Drinking fresh fruit and veggie juice is the fastest way to allow your body to absorb all those vitamins and minerals—even faster than eating the fruits and veggies whole.

FINAL THOUGHTS...

Unfortunately, the conventional treatments for PPP do not have a very high success rate; if you only follow your doctor's recommendations, the chances of achieving remission are slim. My journey to remission wasn't easy; it took extensive research and trial and error before finally getting there. By changing my diet and removing all the stuff that harming my body, I finally regained my health and got my life back.

The way I see it, a healthy diet and a lifestyle change is the only way to heal your PPP. When it comes to autoimmunity, diet works for two reasons:

- It removes foods that cause an autoimmune response and trigger inflammation and antibody activity.

- It floods the body with essential nutrients required for healing.

I tackled my PPP with a shotgun approach. I eliminated as many potentially offending foods, while at the same time as I boosted my immune system, gut healing, and good flora rebuilding. I don't think any one of these changes helped more than the other, but the combination of it all lead to my success.

And in my case, the PPP reversed in just over 90 days, so be patient and stick with it. I also want to mention that during this healing period I kept getting PPP outbreaks, each time on a smaller scale, until they stopped completely.

Troubleshooting problems along the way

In the beginning, I didn't do all the steps – so I didn't get any results. It took a while to apply all these points, and significantly change my diet and lifestyle.

Throughout this journey, I didn't follow a specific diet, but it can be overwhelming in the to figure out what to eat and not to, I therefore recommend you follow either the GAPS, LCHF, FODMAP, Paleo or the anti-candida diet to start off with, until you find the foods that work with your body.

Another piece of advice is to eat the same thing for a full week – the same type of breakfast, the same type of dinner and so on every day for the whole week. Even if it sounds a bit bland, the trade-off is you do not have to worry about what to eat every day. The bonus is you have the whole week planned already.

I can't stress the importance of excluding gluten and sugar during your healing process. Bear in mind all types of carbohydrates turns into sugar in your body when entering the gut, and reducing carbohydrate intake will help.

The hardest part in this journey is to change the way you look at food, as often what previously considered healthy is actually not. One of these big dangers are the low-fat and 'diet' products that are often filled with sugar and flavor enhancers. These sneaky foods are often sold as 'healthy' options. Another misconception is that fat, which we were taught was bad for you, is actually essential for immune system and basic physical functioning.

THE JOURNEY TOWARD REMISSION

Although there will be challenges along the way, my advice is to think about a concrete outcome – how great it will be to walk in nice shoes again, or how you'll feel when you don't need to hide your hands in gloves. Don't try to set a certain date for healing, this, as you know, is ludicrous. Instead, focus on improving your health and making lifestyle changes, one day at a time.

The best way to succeed in healing your PPP is to set a goal, and take baby steps toward it.

The road to healing is both a journey and a destination – it's not a direct route, but, by bringing these changes into your daily life, you will notice an improvement in your health

- **Supplement, supplement**

Invest in good quality supplements. Your body needs good probiotics, zinc, vitamins D3+K2, magnesium, biotin, chlorella, colostrum and colloidal silver water. Give your body what it needs.

- **Cut the crap**

Avoid all processed foods and sugary fizzy drinks. Stop eating sugar. Cut the carbs, and work toward improving gut health. Quitting sugar and taking colloidal silver daily made the biggest difference in healing for me. And, for Pete's sakes, stop eating gluten.

- **Juice it up**

Adopt a daily juicing regime to give your body all the vitamins and minerals it needs to rebuild and heal. Stick with the greens for maximum impact.

- **Get cooking**

Learn how to cook nutritious and healthy meals that don't include gluten and sugar. Check the web for tons of recipes and how-tos.

- **Just say no**

Cut down on alcohol and smoking. Drugs are a definite no-no.

- **Bust the stress**

Find ways to reduce and manage stress. Do something that relaxes you every day – yoga, meditation, calming music, or even just a hot bath. Seriously consider removing the stress triggers in your life (maybe a new job is a good idea after all).

- **Just say yes – to exercise!**

Exercise daily. Go for walks, practice yoga, go swimming. Get active, your body will thank you.

- **Connect with others**

PPP is frustrating, lonely, and isolating. Join online forums on to seek meet others. You'll learn from them and help each other on your journey together – to remission! I frequently visit Inspire for support, which is a forum for people who suffer from all types of psoriasis including palmoplantar pustulosis, the forum is hosted by the National psoriasis foundation in the USA.

The journey to remission takes time, and requires some change on your part. The point is to make the steps so small and manageable that you can check them off relatively quickly and feel a sense of accomplishment. The better you feel, the more motivated you'll be.

Eventually all these steps will be a part of your daily life.

This might sound strange, but in many ways I'm thankful I got sick with PPP. It was my body's way of giving me a wake-up call, and telling me to stop all the harm I was doing to myself.

What makes me most thankful is that PPP is a visible autoimmune disease. By appearing on the skin I was able to realize something is definitely not right, and needed to be dealt with as quickly as possible. Sometimes I think that if I had got cancer instead, it would have been discovered too late, and I might not be here today.

With any autoimmune disease, the path is typically the same – a sad downward spiral. Even with medication, your health deteriorates.

I wanted to share with you my healing journey, and offer you the same solutions. Diet and lifestyle truly can cure all – or at least improve your outcomes.

When faced with chronic illness and autoimmune disorders, unfortunately, there's no quick fix.

Healing is all about the lifestyle you lead. Food, exercise, mindset, and daily stress are all connected, and as long as we live a healing lifestyle, remission will happen.

I hope you reach your final goal of remission. As your health improves, you will regain lost abilities, and your life will become full and beautiful once again.

I wish you all the best in your journey into wellness.

Åsa Kärrman

Resources

1. Women with palmoplantar pustulosis have disturbed calcium homeostasis and a high prevalence of diabetes mellitus and psychiatric disorders: a case-control study.

Eva Hagforsen, Karl Michaëlsson, Ewa Lundgren, Helena Olofsson, Axel Petersson, Alena Lagumdzija, Håkan Hedstrand, Gerd Michaë**lsson**

2. Effects of cigarette smoke exposure on the ultrastructure of the golden hamster parathyroid gland

R. Yano, D. Hayakawa, S. Emura, H. Chen, Y. Ozawa, H. Taguchi and S. Shoumura

Department of Anatomy, Gifu University School of Medicine, Gifu, Japan and

Nursing course, Gifu University School of Medicine, Gifu, Japan

3. Decreased bone mineral density in patients with pustulosis

Nymann P, Kollerup G, Jemec GB, Grossmann E.

4. Dietary phylloquinone and menaquinones intakes and risk of type 2 diabetes.

Beulens JW, van der A DL, Grobbee DE, Sluijs I, Spijkerman AM, van der Schouw YT.

5. Treatments for Chronic Palmoplantar Pustular Psoriasis
A.M. Marsland BSc, MRCP, R.J.G. Chalmers FRCP, and C.E.M. Griffiths MD, FRCP
Dermatology Centre, University of Manchester School of Medicine, Hope Hospital, Manchester, UK

Understanding the immune system

1. http://en.wikipedia.org/wiki/Blood_plasma

2. http://en.wikipedia.org/wiki/Lymph

3. http://en.wikipedia.org/wiki/Thymus

4. The Immune System Cure by Lorn R. Vanderhaeghe and Patrick J.D Bouic, PhD

5. http://www.ncbi.nlm.nih.gov/pmc/articles/PMC1500832/

6. http://www.livescience.com/48482-colon-hydrotherapy-risks-side-effects.html

7. http://www.ncbi.nlm.nih.gov/pubmed/15967639

8. X Zhang, et al. Estrogen effects on Candida albicans: a potential virulence-regulating mechanism. J Infect Dis. 2000 Apr; 181 (4):1441 – 1446. Epub 2000 Apr 13.

9. Cellular and Molecular Biology of Candida albicans Estrogen Response[†]

Georgina Cheng, Kathleen M. Yeater, and Lois L. Hoyer*.

10. https://en.wikipedia.org/wiki/Gluten

12. Gliadin, zonulin and gut permeability: Effects on celiac and non-celiacintestinal mucosa and intestinal cell lines

SANDRO DRAGO1,2, RAMZI EL ASMAR1, MARIAROSARIA DI PIERRO1,2,MARIA GRAZIA CLEMENTE1, AMIT TRIPATHI1, ANNA SAPONE1,MANJUSHA THAKAR, GIUSEPPE IACONO, ANTONIO CARROCCIO,CINZIA D'AGATE, TARCISIO NOT, LUCIA ZAMPINI, CARLO CATASSI &ALESSIO FASANO

13. **Gluten-free Diet in Psoriasis Patients with Antibodies to Gliadin Results in Decreased Expression of Tissue Transglutaminase and Fewer Ki67z Cells in the Dermis**

GERD MICHAEL ÖLSSON, STINA ÅHS, INGRID HAMMARSTRÖM, INGER PIHL LUNDIN and EVA HAGFORSEN

Department of Medical Sciences/Dermatology and Venereology, University Hospital, Uppsala, Sweden

How to Repair a Broken Immune System

1. Silver colloidal nanoparticles: antifungal effect against adhered cells and biofilms of Candida albicans and Candida glabrata

D. R. Monteiro a b , L. F. Gorup c , S. Silva b , M. Negri b , E. R. de Camargo c , R. Oliveira h , D. D. Barbosa a & M. Henriques h

2. https://en.wikipedia.org/wiki/FODMAP

3. https://en.wikipedia.org/wiki/Paleolithic_diet

4. https://en.wikipedia.org/wiki/Low-carbohydrate_diet

5. http://www.the-dermatologist.com/content/insights-treating-palmoplantar-psoriasis

6. Interventions for chronic palmoplantar pustulosis (Review)

Chalmers R, Hollis S, Leonardi-Bee J, Griffiths CEM, Marsland Bsc MRCP A

The Cochrane Collaboration.

7. The role of psychological factors in palmoplantar pustulosis.

Sáez-Rodríguez M[1], Noda-Cabrera A, Alvarez-Tejera S, Guimerá-Martín-Neda F, Dorta-Alom S, Escoda-García M, Fagundo-González E, Sánchez-González R, García-Montelongo R, García-Bustínduy M.

Printed in Great Britain
by Amazon